THE
BODY BALANCE
DIET PLAN

THE
BODY BALANCE
DIET PLAN

LOSE EXCESS WEIGHT, GAIN ENERGY
AND FEEL FANTASTIC
WITH THE SCIENCE OF AYURVEDA

EMINÉ ALI RUSHTON

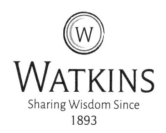

WATKINS
Sharing Wisdom Since
1893

This edition first published in the UK and USA 2015 by
Watkins, an imprint of Watkins Media Limited
19 Cecil Court, London WC2N 4HE

enquiries@watkinspublishing.co.uk

10 9 8 7 6 5 4 3 2 1

Designed and typeset by JCS Publishing Services Limited
Printed and bound in Europe

A CIP record for this book is available from the British Library

ISBN: 978-1-78028-691-4

www.watkinspublishing.com

PUBLISHER'S NOTE
This book is not intended as a replacement for professional medical treatment
and advice. Watkins Media Limited, or any other persons who have been
involved in working on this publication, cannot accept responsibility for any
problem incurred as a result of following any of the advice or recipes in this
work, nor for any errors or omissions, inadvertent or not, that may be found
in the recipes or text. If you are pregnant or breastfeeding or have any special
dietary requirements or medical conditions, it is advisable to consult a medical
professional before following any of the advice or recipes in this book.

Notes on the Recipes
Unless otherwise stated:
• Use medium eggs, fruit and vegetables
• Use fresh ingredients, including herbs and spices
• Do not mix metric and imperial measurements
1 tsp = 5ml   1 tbsp = 15ml   1 cup = 250ml

CONTENTS

FOREWORD

The Body Balance Diet Plan will take you on a journey: a journey of shared experience that allows you to make positive change in your life. It will show you how you can be more informed and more relaxed about who you are – and also about what, how, why and when you eat. It will take you on a journey into the heart of Ayurveda, India's traditional path of healing, so that you can live the life you *want* as much as the life you *need*.

Ayurveda is many things. It is science, it is art, it is poetry and it is practice. Over many generations wise healers have studied the essence of life and how to live. They have created a system that can teach the rest of us how we can fulfil our potential and really live a life full of vitality. They have learned a language of nature that you can easily learn to speak and use in your daily life. And, what's more, it's an amazing and fun experience.

Ayurveda involves understanding that life is dependent on shared relationships, quality and patterns. But it is up to you to weave them together. For example, it is not about how many 'good bacteria' are in your yogurt, but how you digest that yogurt and whether its wet and heavy qualities are right for you. In our busy world it is so easy to get caught up in the latest fad of what is 'good' and what is 'bad' for us. Ayurveda does not pronounce judgement on these things. It is not a moralistic system at all. In fact, it's completely supportive of our natural individuality and idiosyncrasy. Thank goodness! It is a compassionate guide that helps us to understand what we need, how much, and when. You will find this book full of hope and freedom.

One of my teachers told me never to be 'perfectly healthy' because I would only fall off that pinnacle. I should, however, always strive to move toward that goal of perfectly balanced health. He needn't have worried as I am a long way from perfection, but it has inspired me to keep moving in that direction. Ayurveda describes health as being 'comfortable in your self'. Just writing it makes me sit more at ease. Ayurveda will give you the perfect tools to help you understand how to adjust your daily lifestyle according to: how strong your 'digestive fire' is that day, what herbs are best for you, how the weather may affect you that season, what life-stage you are in. Most of all it will help you to be kind to yourself and those you love. It will help you to be perfectly at ease in your self.

Eminé's life-changing experiences can help you find some of that positive change for yourself. By sharing her own journey into how she finds balance, you will get the sense that it is an evolving discovery. And then you have permission to explore; pack what you need for your journey and set out into the wonder of your life. Have an incredible journey.

Sebastian Pole
Co-founder of Pukka Herbs

ACKNOWLEDGEMENTS

It's fair to say that this book didn't 'happen' at the best time. A brand-new baby had just arrived and, with it, this huge deadline. They say it takes a village to raise a child – well, I'd like to thank that village – namely, my inspiring, passionate and true husband and best friend, for being cook, wife, mother, cleaner, comic and even typist when I really ran out of time toward the end. Thanks to my sister, who is always, always there in body and heart, despite being one of the busiest people I know. To my brother who blows me away with his creative fire (his agni!); Natalie, whose balanced work ethic, incredible efficiency and unbelievable generosity got me through a major roadblock – and my beloved mother and father, on either side of my scales, setting the dial at perfect middle, my centre, my balancers, always.

And to the utterly awesome experts I've quizzed and wrangled copy from – who gave their time (and I'm sure sweat and tears) to me, so freely and generously, despite all being incredibly busy people: Annee de Mamiel, with her heart of gold and constancy – what a woman; to Margo Marrone, whose vital, positive company fuels me up for weeks on end and whose generosity of spirit takes my breath away; Selda Enver Goodwin, my soul sister, drawn to what is right and good and empowering like a moral moth to a flame – you inspire me always; the incredibly kind Sunita Passi, whose beauty brand Tri-Dosha inspires me with its authenticity and trueness of vision; Denise Leicester, the soulful, true and pioneering spirit behind Ila Beauty, who also sent my on that first life-changing Ayurvedic retreat to Landaa Giraavaru – thank you, forever; Eve Kalinik, for her humour, sincerity and giddily excited approach to good food – love your RAD spirit. Lastly, Sebastian Pole, a man in the midst of the busiest year of his life, who somehow found time to sit down and write the perfect foreword – so beautiful.

To the kind and wise Vasant Lad for letting me republish his taste table, and to my ever-patient and supportive editors, Sandra Rigby and Fiona Robertson, at Watkins, thank you for the words of encouragement just as my fire petered out . . . they got me over the finish line. And . . . BREATHE.

How to Use this Book

This book is split into nine practical advice-filled chapters, which will simply and quickly teach you every key facet of eating Ayurvedically, to maintain a balanced weight, body and mind. Each chapter explores a different Ayurvedic thread, and it does so with easy-to-follow examples, from tips to boost your digestion, to rituals to help improve your skin. Please take the time to read each chapter, in order, as they'll serve to build a clear and attainable picture of the path you'll be taking. There's a lot to learn, but nothing to fear here – the process is fun, relaxing and eminently beneficial. Once you've read Chapters 1 to 9, you can then embark upon the fantastic immersion diet in Chapter 10, which will prepare you to live Ayurvedically for the first time (or if you've followed Ayurveda before, it is the perfect experience to boost your resolve, reinstate your wellbeing and get you back on the balanced wagon). Chapter 11, then, is filled with varied, interesting and delicious Ayurvedic recipes, which will allow you to eat for your dosha, and begin the exciting process of getting your body to find its own inherent balance.

In the writing of this book I have drawn not only upon my own experiences, but also upon those of several good friends and close colleagues – all of whom used Ayurveda to reshape their lives, and their selves. They, like me, have discovered that once you know your dosha type and the foods that provide your body with its 'dream' fuel, you'll appreciate how good you can feel, and also realize just how much unfounded nonsense lies in a crash, yo-yo or fad diet. Ayurveda is the science of living well, and it's for life.

INTRODUCTION

WELCOME TO THE 'SCIENCE OF LIFE'

It took a life change for me to change my lifestyle.

Having worked in the health and beauty industry for over a decade (I am Beauty and Wellbeing Director at thinking woman's magazine *Psychologies*), I know – without any shadow of a doubt – that crash diets do not work. Dropping a dress size in a week is a recipe for disaster – and makes you more likely to pile those pounds (and more) back on the following month. The only way you can change a yo-yo approach to dieting is to stop fighting your body, and start listening to precisely what it needs – and this is what Ayurveda is all about. It is the very simple but life-changing ability to understand your specific body type, and why it does, and doesn't, do well with certain things. In this book, the focus is on the foods that will heal your body and mind – because Ayurveda believes that food is also medicine. It is a wholly common-sense foundation and works brilliantly for everyone. And of all the 'foundations' I've encountered in my time as an editor, Ayurveda remains the only one that is liveable every single day; it is easy, practical and painless. There is never any deprivation, no hunger, no painful detox side-effects – just a gentle, beautiful, completely natural shift toward a body that is properly understood, and can now thrive.

Despite my long-term interest in this fascinating ancient science, it took me some time to bite. The life change – my first pregnancy – was the jolt I needed to get my body in order despite Ayurveda having been on my radar for years. A few big beauty brands, including the wonderful Aveda, are built on Ayurvedic principles but I had no idea what Ayurveda meant or how to live 'Ayurvedically'. It wasn't until I followed a predominantly Ayurvedic pregnancy plan that I began to see the merit in the way Ayurveda acutely and accurately tunes into, and retunes, your body for the better.

If you've never encountered Ayurveda before – please, bear with me. I realize that some of its words and terms can seem odd. As a wellbeing journalist I often come to things from a cynical perspective; there is, after all, so much nonsense being peddled by 'health' companies. I clearly remember meeting at the start of my career an Ayurveda 'guru' who began talking about doshas and gunas and rasas, and I have to say that it put me off. The entire thing seemed too mystical, and the reality of living 'Ayurvedically' too far removed from my life. The terminology was unfamiliar, the concepts complex and the food seemed to demand a whole new way of living (not to mention a new palate). I felt then that this ancient system was not for me. I was content with my Mediterranean approach to eating and was not inclined to empty and restock my cupboards with strange herbs or to get up early to make barley or quinoa 'kimchi' (a type of porridge) for breakfast.

Still, I was intrigued because there were elements of Ayurveda that struck a chord of truth. It did so because, although I have always eaten healthily – understanding the importance of fresh seasonal fruit and vegetables, and eating food that's as close to nature as possible, by limiting processed foods – I still got colds, felt run-down rather too often, and was always battling eczema. Being told I had too much 'fire' in my system made sense to me – my aforementioned hot and itchy eczema was one thing, but I also got very flustered and antsy in hot weather, and didn't really enjoy spicy food. On a deeper level, I have always been in possession of a temper and also have a strong ambitious fire in my belly. The more I probed this guru, the more he described my intrinsic make-up – from how I dream and sleep, to the way I deal with stress.

He'd worked me out, not because he was supremely intuitive, but because I was an obvious example of a certain dosha type (in my case, Pitta), and he'd seen this type a thousand times before. I went away with this word 'Pitta' in my head, and it wasn't until years later, at the launch of an Ayurvedic beauty brand, where I was once again told that I was Pitta, that I started to think there might be something in this. At around the same time I became pregnant, and my real Ayurvedic journey properly began.

I have never restricted calories or followed a 'diet book'. Eating Ayurvedically and healthily is not 'going on a diet' – it's about wellbeing. Upon getting pregnant, my overwhelming fear of childbirth led me to seek out the advice of the Ayurvedic expert Dr

Gowri Motha – the author of *The Gentle Birth Method*. A couple of my friends had followed her plan and had had good births. Others were less enthusiastic (such is the unpredictable nature of childbirth) but I thought I'd give it a whirl. I had nothing to lose. Despite not following her advice to the letter, I did incorporate a great deal of the Ayurvedic dietary recommendations into my 40 weeks and ended up having a very speedy, medicine- and intervention-free natural birth. While no birth is easy, I was one of the lucky ones and I was sure that my immediate physical recovery owed a lot to the approach I'd taken. This programme – which had led me to gain just a stone in total during the pregnancy – was determined by the ancient Indian 'science of life', the traditional system of medicine: Ayurveda.

I – just like you are about to – began that journey by determining my dosha – my unique body and personality 'type'. Understanding this has allowed me to work out how and what to eat to maximize my energy and, crucially, shift the uncomfortable excess weight that can so often creep on during the course of our mostly sedentary lives. As a journalist, I spend about 50 per cent of my week sat in front of a computer, so despite having had a wonderful birth, immediate recovery and easy weight loss as I breastfed, my weight increased after my return to work. I was also hugely sleep-deficient, trapped in that classic exhausted energy-low and sugar-high cycle that I adopted in a bid to get me through my working day, often on less than three hours' sleep. It was not a good time! The powerful Ayurvedic system I was able to embrace while pregnant sadly fell by the wayside once I returned to work, and the sleepless fog took over. This was not because Ayurvedic living would have been difficult to maintain, but because I had not yet explored the ways in which Ayurveda can be easily, practically and realistically woven into the fabric of our busy, chaotic, modern lives. It's hard to look back and see just how much my family and I would have benefited from Ayurveda at that crucial time, but we live and we learn – and that's what this book is all about.

It was not until my first daughter was 18 months old that I found the strength and opportunity to get myself back on track – at the extraordinary Spa and Ayurvedic Retreat at Four Seasons Landaa Giraavaru, in the Maldives – where I arrived sleep-deficient, sluggish and in possession of too many pounds, and left a week later, a lot lighter in both body and mind. Determining your dosha is just the beginning – it is the start of a life-long lesson in how your body works, what balances and imbalances it, why you regularly crave certain things, and how to eat to ensure that your metabolism is permanently switched on at an optimal level.

What is Ayurveda – and Why Does it Work for us Today?

Ayurveda is the most ancient comprehensive system of medicine – it is believed to date from around 3000 BCE. While its principles can appear simplistic, once you start to practise them it's impossible to doubt their relevance. But, clearly we've come a very long way in 5,000 years, which is why I would never want to swallow the Ayurvedic textbook whole. What I do passionately believe is just how astute the Ayurvedic consultation can be, and how it remains the only holistic way in which to treat the body. Today we might go and see a doctor, who prescribes drugs, then a homeopath who gives us alternative medicine, an acupuncturist who works on pressure points and meridians, a personal trainer to lose weight or get fit, or a masseur who helps us relax . . . the ways in which we seek help for our health issues are diverse – no one practitioner is able to offer us a 360-degree health solution. Every expert is an expert in something specific, be it general medicine, homeopathy, aromatherapy or dermatology, but when we have a rash, a bad stomach, can't sleep, get back-ache and are overweight – where do we go first? The GP? And then when the pills or creams don't work – where from there?

The beauty of Ayurveda is that it applies a scientific approach to living. In Sanskrit *ayu* means 'life' and *veda* means 'science', so, how to live sensibly, healthily and be in possession of the knowledge of life are all meanings that we can take from the word Ayurveda itself.

Ayurveda embraces all aspects of wellbeing, including our spiritual health – something, sadly, that is so often overlooked by Western medical practitioners. Ayurveda counts health not just as physical wellbeing, but also as a state of uninterrupted physical, mental and spiritual happiness and fulfilment. Now, isn't that a much nicer way to think of 'good health'?

When our minds and bodies are imbalanced we see the inevitable consequences. With the incidence of stress-related ailments continually on the rise (Bupa estimates an average of 10.5 million working days are lost in the UK, every year, to stress-related illness), it makes sense to try to solve the underlying problem. When your gut isn't working optimally, a lot can go wrong. Immunity is compromised, sleep is affected, we are not vital, we do not feel strong, we are not firing on all cylinders. It's pretty common-sense stuff.

Ayurveda stems from ancient Vedic science – it is the medical arm of the Vedic system, which also incorporates yoga, meditation and even astrology. And, while I am not suggesting you become a star-sign addict any time soon, I would absolutely vouch for the benefits of practising meditation and yoga alongside following the Body Balance Diet.

This book is a plan for life – not just for the days prior to squeezing into your swimwear – and I hope that once you feel and see the benefits, you'll want to incorporate more and more elements into your life on a daily basis. To this end, I've also asked several great friends, all of whom are experts in their alternative health fields, to share their best advice with you.

Ayurveda is, and always has been, about the treatment of the individual as a 'whole'. And if you want to feel that wholeness, that sense of centre, that feeling of balance, there's no better way to do it than by following the holistic expertise throughout this book, from seasonal cues and clues from revered expert Annee de Mamiel to essential healthy living tips from the Organic Pharmacy's inspiring co-founder Margo Marrone.

Throughout the book I have sought to balance my professional experience as a wellbeing editor with a decade's personal experience. I have drawn on trusted alternative practices (such as aromatherapy) while also basing my principles on a foundation of solid, modern, medical sense. We know a lot more today than we did 5,000 years ago, so I feel it's remiss to ignore the enormous progress we've made in health and wellbeing, which is why I cite modern studies on health and nutrition. Fascinatingly, Ayurveda almost always nails it and has a pertinent answer for every health concern I've ever encountered. Ayurveda deems that food is medicine – a belief that we're only now embracing again, as we become privy to the effects that decades of fast, convenience and junk food have had on our bodies. People knew then that everything they put into their bodies had an effect, good or bad, and made a rich healing science from this knowledge.

I hope you enjoy the process: savour the food, enjoy the sense of renewed energy, delight in the newfound sense of peace that will come when your body is balanced . . . that's the thing about Ayurveda – at some point or another the spiritual side of the science takes hold, and you begin to feel different.

Why a Balanced Body is a Slim Body

I believe in Ayurveda, but I also realize that this ancient science may, for some, require a leap of faith. Accepting that just because you have identified your body type, and have learned what and how to eat in a bid to best support that type – and that this simple knowledge will then bring about enormous changes to your wellbeing – well, it can seem too good to be true. I felt that way during my first immersion diet – but soon I also felt wonderful.

> **The Ayurvedic Principles for Balancing Your Body**
>
> Eat according to your body's personality, its **dosha** type, to balance the elements: ether, air, fire, water and earth (Chapter 2)
>
> Eat a balance of the different tastes, **rasas**, to match your body type (Chapter 3)
>
> Eat in the right way and at the right time to balance your digestive fire, **agni** (Chapter 4)
>
> Eat simple combinations of food that are easily digestible (Chapter 5)
>
> Eat seasonally to enjoy the best foods and balance the elements of each season (Chapter 6)
>
> Eat food that helps balance your personality trait, your **guna** (Chapter 7)

Within just a few days I could tell my body was responding well to the 'perfect match' food I was consuming, but I didn't realize that weight loss would follow suit. Yet it did – eight pounds dropped off in a week. Bizarre, because I'd done little exercise (aside from a couple of short snorkel sessions) and hadn't been very active at all (as with most beach holidays, I spent most of it in the shade, snoring to the sound of the sea). I'd simply eaten differently, according to my dosha type – but still eaten well, with a comforting breakfast, a three-course lunch, and a lighter dinner most days. Food was varied, fresh and seasonal. I'd eaten slowly, chewing well, breathing well as I ate, because I was relaxed to the point of somnolence for the first time in a long, long time (my first baby didn't sleep well!). Because my body was relaxed, my levels of cortisol, the stress hormone that tends to disrupt sleep and metabolism, were low for the first time in 18 months. The food I was eating was fuelling my metabolism and keeping my digestive fire – *agni* – optimal. But, I wondered, would the weight go back on the moment I returned to normal life, with all its stresses, strains and time constraints?

The answer is, no, but with conditions. And those conditions involved changing certain things about the way I lived, to ensure I would have time to eat better food, in a better way, most of the time. I sought out a couple of Ayurvedic cafés close to my workplace, but I could also have food that worked for me from my local salad bar (which served great seasonal stews and soups), and I got into the habit of cooking far more, too. I have an advantage on the home cooking front in that my husband is a wonderful cook, and also an Ayurvedic convert – indeed, many of the recipes in this book are thanks to his passion, flair and experimentation.

The changes first involved a bit of alteration to my routine and to the way we prepared, spiced and ate our food, but the biggest change came from the way the right food correlates with feeling 'right'. Because Ayurveda is a complete science, the food you eat is medicine in itself. It is not a short cut to a dip in the scales. The weight loss happens, but it happens steadily, naturally, in an unforced way – and the brilliance is that it stays that way.

This is because when you embark upon the immersion diet (see Chapter 10), which ought to be the starting point for everyone beginning an Ayurvedic journey, your body is being reawakened; its metabolism is being properly fired up for the first time in a long time, and the latent fat and toxins within your body (which it has not had a chance to expel, so busy is it with digesting the daily menu and keeping you upright) are finally exorcised. This build-up of toxins – caused by improper diet, pollution and stress – which we carry around with us every day is called *ama*.

If you're one of those people who is relatively thin all over, but has stubborn stomach, thigh or bottom fat, Ayurveda says there's a reason for this. That reason is that some of the body's toxic detritus is water-soluble and is lost more easily with diet and exercise, as you sweat, and as you excrete naturally. The rest of your ama is held within your fat cells, which are most commonly deposited around this mid-section. In Ayurveda, we're told that these fat cells are continually swollen. When we put on weight, it's these fat cells expanding further due to our improper diet; it's insoluble fat being stored in increasing amounts. A crash diet will help us shift other fat, but not this fat – the stubborn fat that never goes anywhere.

Getting to a point where you shift the ama that's stored within your adipose tissue is not extreme. Nothing in Ayurveda is extreme, which is why I adore it so wholeheartedly. The process is natural and simple (you won't be sick or feel unwell or faint – all things you may have heard about or experienced on other 'diets' or extreme detoxes) and as you read on, you'll discover all you need to know about Ayurveda's gentle but ever so powerful way of bringing your body into balance, naturally.

From an Ayurvedic stance, our modern lifestyle appears to be utterly counter-intuitive. We often skip breakfast (or have a cup of coffee, which escalates our Pitta dosha (see Chapter 2) and promotes yet more build-up of ama), we grab a less-than-satisfying lunch and eat it too quickly (which will not do your digestive fire, or agni, any good), then we return home, exhausted, and gorge on food that can't be properly digested because our agni is at its lowest ebb, which sends ama soaring, and those fat stores building yet again.

Getting balanced, and getting your body back on track, requires the realization that the answer to your 'why can't I lose weight' question might well be 'all of the above' – you're not at the weight you want to be because your body is struggling with your lifestyle, as so many of our bodies are as we rush from A to B with barely a breath in between.

Once you've understood this, and have gone on to make the necessary changes outlined throughout this book, these ways of eating will become second nature – likewise, slim, vital and motivated will become second nature. With Ayurveda I have learned what it means for my body to be balanced, what it actually feels like to be lighter and leaner and healthier. I have also learned that you can bring about great change in your body without pain, trauma or deprivation. It's life-changing, it really is.

one

WHY THE BODY BALANCE DIET IS DIFFERENT

As soon as you begin scanning the recipes, and reading the food principles of the Body Balance Diet Plan, you'll immediately notice some very clear and distinct differences between this and other diets. It is based on six common-sense principles.

1. 'All Protein' is All Wrong

Unlike the Dukan, Atkins and South Beach diets, the Body Balance Diet is *not* all about protein. It centres on whole grains and vegetables, hammering home the truth that, in themselves, *carbohydrates do not make you fat*. There are three types of carbohydrates: sugar, starch and fibre. There is nothing wrong with any of these (fruit, milk and vegetables contain 'sugar', and consuming this is not comparable to eating teaspoons of refined white sugar – we are also getting important vitamins, minerals and antioxidants from these foods) and it's impossible to eat a balanced diet without them. Starchy and fibre-rich carbohydrates include mineral-rich pulses and beans, grains and cereals; these are essential for the release of energy and they're also low in calories while being filling. The basis for many Ayurvedic dishes is a mixture of pulses/beans and vegetables (think of traditional lentil or chickpea vegetable curries) – delicious, satisfying and healthy.

Without the all-important fibre from complex carbohydrates, such as whole grains, pulses/beans and some vegetables, the food we put into our bodies will not pass through our systems efficiently. Indeed, if you've ever tried a protein-only diet, you've probably experienced the constipation that comes with it.

While I am a big lover and enjoyer of omega-rich fish, organic chicken, goat's and ewe's cheeses – and generally eat a lot more protein than strict Ayurvedic eaters do – I do not need to eat animal protein at every single meal. My diet does, however, contain a variety of 'hidden' proteins (found in some foods that you might expect to be classed as 'carbs'): namely buckwheat, hemp and chia, which are all ostensibly 'grains' but are in fact complete proteins (called 'pseudocereals'). They're a great thing to eat if you are vegetarian, and help ensure your diet includes all of the essential amino acids that our bodies can't make for themselves and must therefore gain from what we eat. Quinoa too is a complete protein, and also high in fibre, phosphorous, iron and magnesium, while being gluten free. Quinoa can be the dullest ingredient going, but be inventive with it, or load the food that accompanies it with tons of flavour (as I have done in the recipes at the back of this book), and you'll soon become partial to it, and love how conveniently fast it is to cook (it also freezes and defrosts well if dinner needs to be on the table quickly).

2. Stop the Vicious Cycle, without Being Too Virtuous

The Body Balance Diet Plan is not a diktat. One of the most important wellbeing lessons is that continual denial and deprivation are the surest routes to failure and weight issues. I eat very well – I would never dream of going hungry – which means I never obsess about food. When I am hungry, my tummy may rumble, or energy levels wane, and I sit down to eat a delicious meal, always eating whatever I fancy at the time, knowing that in so doing I'll feel satisfied afterwards and a lot less likely to look for quick-fix treats to deliver that absent satiety.

I will eat any food group, I will have some sugar, but I do not eat 'fake' food that's laden with horrible health-sapping additives. If I check a label and see more E numbers than recognizable words, I leave it. If I see sulphites and hydrogenates, I leave it. I eat burgers and fries and ice cream, but these are burgers and fries I make myself and simple organic ice cream from the supermarket with no chemical additives. Because of this I think my body craves nutritious food. I believe that once we begin eating well, and understand what it is to feel satisfied and nourished by every meal, the body can finally balance itself – and blood sugar is a part of this. So often, we grab that chocolate bar or cookie because we're suddenly hungry and have nothing else to hand. But, if we prepare ahead, we won't get caught out. I use the leftovers from dinner – maybe roasted veg, salmon, chicken or lentils – and create a quick super salad by adding fresh leaves, cucumber and olives. I put it all into a Tupperware box that night, ready to take to work with me the next morning. Or I'll simply take the leftovers as they come – whether it's curry, soup or a tortilla. Cooking a bit extra is a good thing if you get into a habit of taking leftovers for lunch the next day. It's certainly made my life easier (and healthier). I also try to carry some form of healthy snack on me at all times – a piece of fruit, perhaps, or one of my Chia Choc Bars (see pages 212–13) – to ensure that if I get caught out without time for a proper meal, I can at least eat something wholesome that will not send my blood sugar spiralling (which may in turn kick off a vicious sugary snack cycle!).

Being inventive is also a key part of staying satisfied. Food should be rich with flavour (and learning about the six tastes will reinvigorate your life and your palate), seasonal and exciting. Ayurveda excels here, as you'll see!

3. Trust Your Body

Of late, the way we eat seems to have a lot less to do with what we actually want, and more to do with what we've been led to believe we *ought* to want. Most people will have a rough idea of what constitutes 'healthy eating' – yet, more people than ever are now succumbing to deprivation-based diets. Having worked for a long time in magazine offices full of people who seem to be on permanent diets, I've lost count of the number of times colleagues have compared the calories of their lunches and deemed everything from grapes to goat's cheese 'evil'.

What has struck me, again and again, is how gullible the dieting masses are. And how keenly dieters seem to set aside common sense in the pursuit of a very quick fix. Calorie counting is, in my book, a problem. Why? Because it overrides common sense and assumes we must live by a very simplistic equation. Women assume they need around 2,000 calories a day, men 2,500, yet we are all individuals, made up of differing ratios of different materials (fat, muscle, water), and as such, we all require a different calorie intake. Our metabolisms differ; we may be sedentary or very active; we may or may not have allergies and intolerances . . . the list goes on. The moment we trust the calories on the packet before we trust ourselves, we have a problem. I don't mind that the homemade banana bran muffin I enjoy possesses what any dieting person would deem to be too many calories. I know that it is low in refined sugar and made with coconut oil, a far superior fat to 'fake' refined margarine (it has also been shown that coconut oil can increase good HDL cholesterol in the blood and restore normal thyroid function). I know it's good for me. I know my body likes it and, by god, I know I enjoy eating it. So I'll have it all, and won't waste a single moment weighing it and calculating whether I should feel guilty.

I believe that if you trust yourself to make the right food decisions, your body will find its happy weight, completely account – then you take away that awful, sense-robbing panic that can make us fear food.

A friend said she would spend all morning nervous with fear about what to have for lunch, and then was depressed all afternoon at having made the wrong decision. How exhausting! Even after paying for a personal trainer for several years, my friend never managed to maintain a healthy weight. A drop was often followed – and swiftly, to boot – by another, bigger, gain. Why? Because her chaotic food confusion had gone on to confuse her body. Her body didn't know when the next meal would arrive, or where it would come from; whether it would be entirely devoid of nutritional value (the classic 'I've not eaten all week, so I'm going to treat myself to two pots of ice cream' mentality), or too small to cause even a ripple in her already-flagging metabolism. As a result, her body was living in permanent starvation mode. During the weeks when my friend trained for several hours a night and ate next to nothing, she would be frustrated to tears in seeing no shift whatsoever in the scales.

What I saw in my friend was someone who knew so much about 'dieting' that she knew nothing about eating. Someone who trusted the black-and-white rules in every book so much that she utterly distrusted herself, and her own instincts. Someone who feared food so actively, it made her very ill, and very stressed – and more overweight than ever. Food was not to be enjoyed, but to be measured, weighed and avoided for as long as humanly possible – and then, ultimately, gorged upon, once hunger and desperation and self-hatred got the better of her. It is heartbreaking, and the most vicious cycle of all.

5. Adapt your Menu to your Lifestyle

Consider this: 'Breakfast like a king and dine like a pauper'. I'll admit, I swore by it. Until I realized that I always suffered a post-breakfast energy slump and noon sugar-craving spike on days when I'd had a right royal feast at the start of the day. It took me a few months of trial and error before I understood that my ideal breakfast was somewhat lighter than I'd grown used to. Instead of a large bowl of cereal, or two thick slices of wholemeal toast with peanut butter and jam, on my Ayurvedic immersion I rotated fresh fruit, goat's yogurt with sweet berries, a light millet and pear porridge (see pages 174–6) and eggs (sometimes whites only) on spelt toast almost every morning for a week. It left me feeling more satisfied and energized than I had been when eating a more 'filling' breakfast. Often, the intense 'hunger' we feel upon waking is actually thirst. If you drink a large glass of warm water as soon as you wake, you'll be able to gauge that your digestive fire (agni) is not overly strong. Lighter breakfasts are easier on the stomach – our bodies are waking up, remember – but they're also less taxing on energy levels. Digesting any food requires energy, so we can only comfortably eat larger meals when our digestive fire is optimal, and won't overly tax our bodies in the process.

For this reason, a lighter breakfast and larger lunch is optimal. But, because I have to adapt Ayurvedic wisdom to my own modern-world routine when I often have breakfast meetings around 9am, I will wake and have a large glass of hot water and a piece of ripe fruit around 7am, which gets my digestive fire stoked, and then enjoy a good breakfast a couple of hours later (favourites include eggs and smoked salmon, porridge or kedgeree) during my meeting. At 1pm I will then sit down to a simpler lunch – some soup, a small bowl of stew, a warm seasonal salad. This means I don't have any huge dips in energy because meals are evenly spaced, and also means I don't overtax my digestive system with too much to eat too early on in the day.

During my immersion I also proved my long-held belief that watermelon is a bit of a miracle food. Being of Cypriot heritage, I've spent more summers than I can count on this sun-drenched island, where my breakfasts always revolve around the ruby-red watermelon. Enjoyed in wedges with lightly salted grilled/broiled halloumi, drunk first thing as a fresh juice, accompanied by a clutch of salty black olives, or simply eaten alongside toast and local honey, watermelon is one of those amazing foods that gets the body working more efficiently. It is a phenomenal hydrator – being 97 per cent water. Dr Howard Murad's book *The Water Secret* explains that when you get your water from food, it has a big impact and the cells absorb the water more efficiently, quenching your thirst more effectively than drinking glass after glass of water. I craved watermelon like a lunatic while I was pregnant, and now my children love it too.

So, in short, I went from being a life-long big breakfast eater to a morning grazer. I learned another lesson along the way: you cannot change your body, or your energy, until you have learned its language.

6. Don't Eat What You Don't Like

During my Ayurvedic immersion I learned a great deal about myself. Even when I am hungry I cannot force myself to eat something I do not enjoy. At the retreat, not all of the food was to my liking. I have spent too long having a bowl of cereal or peanut butter on toast for breakfast to switch to spiced mung bean curry at 7am! So, I sat down with the doctor leading the retreat and explained that, although the curry would have made a lovely lunch, I just could not stomach it for breakfast. He explained that it's better to be relaxed and eat well than to panic and eat nothing. So, rather than going hungry – hunger, is as I have already said, the surest route to diet failure – I wandered down to the buffet, served myself some eggs, then a spelt crois-sant with honey, and enjoyed another glass of watermelon juice. Although it was not the Ayurvedic breakfast, I felt absolutely no guilt. It was what I wanted that day. It tasted delicious. I enjoyed it. Did it set my 'diet' back? No, not at all. Because the breakfast I really wanted paved the way to my wholesome lunch, and a lighter dinner.

The next day, I ate the Ayurvedic breakfast of lightly poached pears and grain porridge, had a lighter lunch, and after an hour's snorkelling and a long beach walk before sunset, returned to my room to see a very small bowl of vegetable soup for dinner. Now, I know Ayurveda traditionalists encourage a light dinner . . . but . . . it left me wanting. The moment I wanted, I began to wonder what was in my mini-bar, and that chocolate bar that had been left there began to look more and more attractive. So yet again,

I looked back over the foods my dosha gets on best with, and ordered some lentil kebabs and a fresh green salad. Tasty, filling and good for me – unlike that chocolate bar! And when it came to my weigh-in at the end of the week: well, what can I say – no hunger, no pain, no headaches, no withdrawal or denial, and a still a loss of eight pounds.

When you do not deny yourself, you become calm and collected around food. You begin to make the right decisions rather than being swept along in a chain reaction of all the wrong ones.

Your body will find its balance – if you trust it to do so.

So, there you have it – the six common-sense principles that underlie the Body Balance Diet. Next, determining your dosha type.

two

DETERMINE YOUR DOSHA TYPE (AND WHY YOU ARE THE WAY YOU ARE)

Ayurveda is based on the beautifully simple principle of seeking balance. I do realize, however, that modern life is not always conducive to a balanced sense of being. I can vouch for it on a personal level, with two young children and several strings to the working bow. I'm often pulled in so many different directions I literally lose my balance – clumsiness, for me, is always because of having too little time, not enough care. It's a sign to stop, whatever you're doing: just STOP. Breathe in. Breathe out. In again. Then pick up where you left off, calmer, more carefully. Identifying those moments of short-breath-inducing panic – I'm late! I'm tired! I'm stressed! – are key – you have to recognize them and tackle them. Otherwise they will overwhelm every moment, every day, and before you know it you're living in a constant state of exhaustion and anxiety.

Ayurveda is, therefore, in many ways, the perfect tonic for our incredibly hectic modern lives. Even if you're busy, stressed, overwhelmed, the simple act of eating Ayurvedically will help to keep your body in balance in a way that will strengthen it against the day's challenges. It's the best starting point for busy people, because it gently, very gently, brings the body into line without shocking the system. You can still go about your business, still be productive and driven, but feeling far better, calmer, happier and healthier than you did before. You'll be stronger, you'll sleep better, you'll feel lighter and more energized, you'll feel yourself again.

This chapter is about discovering your individual body 'personality' – and now, your Ayurvedic journey can really begin!

Ayurveda is based on the theory that all living and non-living things are made up of five *elements*. We cannot see the five elements, but we can understand them because of what they do within our own bodies.

The Five Elements

ETHER, AIR, FIRE, WATER and EARTH

To explain the way these elements function, Ayurveda has divided them into three entities, called *doshas*.

The Three Doshas

VATA – which is predominantly Ether and Air
PITTA – which is predominantly Fire and Water
KAPHA – which is predominantly Water and Earth

Everyone possesses all three doshas – we need to in order to carry out all the different functions of our body. But the doshas make up different proportions within each of us – and this proportion allows us to calculate our specific dosha type. This is your *prakruti* – a sanskrit word for our constitution that also means 'first creation'. Essentially, this is the body type you were born with, it is your inherent nature, and it does not change. Eating according to your prakruti – which the chart on pages 28–9 will help you do – will ensure that you stay balanced. We can lose or gain weight, run marathons or sit still, learn everything or nothing, be old, young or in between . . . but this fundamental constitution will not change. Poetic, isn't it?

If you would like to learn more about *vikriti*, which is the way an imbalance shows up within our bodies when we are not living according to our nature (very common in modern life!), visit www.balanceplan.co.uk for further reading.

Determine Your Dosha Type

Look at the chart below, and choose the statement in each row that most applies to you

	Vata	Pitta	Kapha
Body build	Thin light frame Prominent bones and veins Difficult to gain weight	Medium frame Constant weight Easy to lose and gain weight	Strong with excellent stamina or heavy and stocky. Difficult to lose weight
Skin	Dry, lack of tone or lustre May flake or chap	Combination skin, lustrous complexion, oily t-zone, prone to blackheads, rashes or pigmentation	Radiant skin, prone to shine, thick and resilient, oily appearance
Hair	Dry, dull, split ends	A combination – moderately oily, but also prone to thinness or bald spots	Shiny hair, oily scalp, looks glossy and grows easily
Nails	Dry, may be brittle. cracked, thin or splitting	Pink, soft, medium strength and rate of growth	Thick, white and shiny
Perspiration	Sweat little	Sweat a lot	Sweat moderately
Appetite	Varies – sometimes strong, sometimes weak; irregular eating habits and patterns	Strong and sharp – does not like to miss meals (and gets irritable if does so); excellent digestion	Constant, but can be weak in the morning; may skip breakfast
Digestion	Occasional gas and bloating	Occasional acidity and heartburn	Occasional heartburn and nausea
Bowel movements	Prone to constipation (stools less than once a day)	Prone to loose bowels at least once a day	Regular movements – at least once a day

	Vata	Pitta	Kapha
Sleep	Light sleep – six hours average Prefers afternoon naps	Moderate – seven hours average Sleeps soundly in short bursts	Sound and heavy – likes to wake late Feels slow after morning or afternoon naps
Weather	Does not like cold weather Adores sun and likes to 'bask' Poor circulation – often has cold hands and feet	Does not like very hot or sunny weather Remains in the shade, uses lots of SPF and avoids over-exposure	More tolerant to weather extremes than others Uncomfortable with cold or damp weather
Activity	Quick movements, speedy actions Energy comes in bursts, followed by sudden bouts of fatigue	Moderately active Lots of energy, does not tire easily	Slow in movements, can be lazy Not inclined to 'get up and go'
Positive personality traits	Energetic, enthusiastic, creative, flexible; takes initiative; lively conversationalist	Powerful intellect, good concentration; a good decision-maker, speaker and teacher; ambitious, passionate, authoritative; expresses emotions in a strong and clear way	Calm, thoughtful, comfortable with routine, loyal, patient, steady and supportive, firm in decisions, down to earth; does not overreact
Negative personality traits	When stressed may get overly anxious or irrepressibly worried; indecisive and easily influenced	Aggressive; when stressed can be short-tempered or argumentative	When stressed can be very stubborn and resistant to change; depressed, avoids difficult people and situations

Add up the number of statements you've marked in each column: Vata, Pitta or Kapha.

The column that has the largest number of statements that apply to you is your majority dosha, which tends to work alongside your second largest number, your minority dosha.

It's rare for people to be very clearly one single dosha type.

Most people are obviously bi-dosha. I, for example, scored 1 Vata, 8 Pitta and 4 Kapha. I am predominantly Pitta, but Kapha is significant. This makes me Pitta–Kapha. But, as all living things are made up of all five elements, we need all three doshas for our body to function, so there is some Vata in me too.

Predominantly Vata Types Are . . .

. . . naturally slender – these types find it hard to gain weight and can lose weight very easily through stress, illness and worry. You're drawn to creative and spiritual pursuits – many yoga teachers, singers and dancers are Vata types. You're naturally generous, kind and sensitive, and can also be intuitive, but when imbalanced you're nervy and fidgety; you often find it hard to sit still and must always keep yourself occupied.

You are a fast talker – you've probably been called a chatterbox more than once! The restlessness within you drives your creative endeavours; you want to try to experience as much as you can, and are very enthusiastic about life. Vata can also make you prone to constipation, or the opposite, loose bowels. You are not a deep sleeper and tend to have vivid dreams, but slip in and out of sleep, and feel just fine on as little as five or six hours a night. You can be drawn to high-impact sport, but will find that soothing meditative sports are better for you – yoga is ideal, though not the more active power forms. You really do feel the cold and suffer with poor circulation. You always dream of being on a hot beach somewhere, and are continually craving warmth, which nurtures and balances your body. You can suffer with weak nails, dry skin and coarse, brittle hair. You don't sweat a lot. Bone and back problems plague this dosha type. You're a fast learner but can also forget just as quickly, and though you're very driven toward new adventures and experiences you can have weak willpower. The focus for balancing Vata types must be on foods that warm, soothe, calm, hydrate and nourish.

Predominantly Pitta Types Are . . .

. . . quite easy to spot. You're the driven types who can stand up in front of others and speak very assertively and charismatically – getting to the point quickly. You have a real fire in your belly, which, on the positive side, makes you a high achiever, a strong leader and successful in business. When imbalanced, though, you can be angry, aggressive, intolerant and insensitive to others.

Pitta types can think the world revolves around them and need reminding that others have feelings too! Your appetite for everything – food, sex, sleep – is high. You live a full life, but also need to recoup that energy at night, with a solid seven hours (more and you'll feel sluggish and 'off'). Heat aggravates Pitta – you need cooling down, not heating up – so you can get very irritable and flustered in summer, prone to sweating copiously,

31

and also producing strong sharp body odour. Pitta types do better in cooler climes. You've got good strong digestion but, if imbalanced, you are prone to diarrhoea (you also produce more urine and sweat than other dosha types). When digestion is out of sync, heartburn, reflux and painful indigestion are all common. Pitta types are balanced by cooling foods.

Predominantly Kapha Types Are . . .

. . . well built and strong. 'Big boned' often describes the Kapha type. Your body is beautifully nourished and this also shows in your skin, hair and nails, which tend to be smooth, shiny and glossy. Your appetite is steady – you like to enjoy larger meals, but your metabolism can be slow.

You enjoy sleep. Like a cat curled up by the fire, you like to take your time, and often feel you need time to be still, rest and do nothing (the opposite of Vata types, who feel they must always be busy, occupied and mobile). You like your creature comforts, and you are a wonderfully loyal, trustworthy, calm and steady individual, so you make a wonderful parent. Many of the most successful people within our society are Kapha types – their unerring compassion and quiet confidence make them do well.

You have great stamina and, when you push yourself, you are often surprised by what you can achieve. Naturally, you tend toward low-impact exercise, like walking. Food-wise, Kapha types have very strong cravings for sweet and fatty foods, which hinders their metabolism further and can make weight gain inevitable. Kapha types are most likely to suffer diet-related disorders such as diabetes and obesity, but are also prone to allergies and asthma. Kapha types need energizing and drying foods that will elevate digestion and kickstart metabolism.

And now that you know your dosha type, you've been given the key to finding life-long balance within your body. From this point onward, you'll discover which foods work best for your dosha and why, and how eating according to your dosha can transform your life, affecting everything from your mood to your sleeping patterns.

Your dosha – Vata, Pitta or Kapha – can be managed by the foods that you eat. Being balanced is always your goal – and in Ayurveda, that means achieving as equal a balance of the three doshas, Vata, Pitta and Kapha, as possible. So if you are mostly Vata, you do not want to increase Vata any more, meaning that you'll need to eat foods that increase Pitta and Kapha. If you are mostly Pitta, you want to eat foods that raise Vata and Kapha, reducing Pitta. And so it goes on. It's a slightly unusual way to think of things – one might assume if you are Vata you should eat Vata-boosting foods – but, again, just keep taking your mind back to the idea of balance, and your body as a set of weighing scales. Every meal you eat is about bringing the needle of the scales to the optimal middle – where every element is equal and constant. If you're tri-doshic, and all three doshas are on a similar footing within your constitution, you're one of the lucky ones as you're inherently more balanced. You tend to have a robust body and rarely get ill, you're adaptable and resilient. Because the three doshas are already present in you in relatively equal amounts, imbalance for you most often stems from your environment. So, it's crucial to eat seasonally, to ensure your body gets foods that pacify the imbalanced dosha naturally – an example of this would be eating more spicy, warming foods in winter, when your Kapha will elevate. Yes, it's mainly common sense!

By eating more of the tastes that pacify your dosha, you'll be balancing your body.

You can now move on to Chapter 3 and learn about the six tastes.

three

WHAT TO EAT: THE SIX TASTES AND WHY YOU CRAVE THEM

We instinctively crave variety in our diets. It's our bodies' way of trying to ensure we get all the things we need: a balance of proteins, carbohydrates, fats, vitamins, minerals and amino acids. We may not always be aware of why we want to eat the way we do, but even when grabbing a cheese-and-tomato sandwich and bag of salt-and-vinegar crisps/potato chips, we're instinctively looking to tick off as many flavours and textures as possible: you've got that creamy butter, sweet bread, milky cheese, the sour tomatoes and vinegar, the salty tang, and don't forget the crunch of the crisps beside the soft squidge of the bread. I'm one of those people who always fancies a crunchy snack with a sandwich, and I also don't like eating a salad without something silken or creamy on top – be it goat's cheese, feta, tofu, a dollop of hummus or some juicy chicken breast. I feel that every meal needs to satisfy, and it can only do that if it ticks off all the right flavour and texture boxes.

In Ayurveda there are six tastes (known as *rasas*).

The Six Rasas

SWEET, SOUR, SALTY, BITTER, ASTRINGENT and PUNGENT

The rasas cover every single food out there, though it's not always immediately obvious which foods fall into which categories (meat and dairy are classified as Sweet, for example). Some rasas are better for your dosha than others. This is because each taste, or rasa, is made up of two of the same five elements that also make up the doshas – Earth, Fire, Water, Ether and Air. You will shortly learn that if you are, for example, Kapha (and primarily Earth and Water elements), then you will therefore need to eat fewer Earth and Water tastes (that would be fewer Sweet, Sour and Salty, and more Bitter, Pungent and Astringent foods). It is always about balance – eating more of the elements your body doesn't naturally possess, and fewer of the things it's already inherently rich in. So, for cold, damp Kapha that means eating hot, spicy, drying, warming foods. This will all become explicit and clear as you read this chapter, and now that you know your dosha type, you can work out which tastes should make up the bulk of your diet. There's my Rasa Cheatsheet on page 39 to help with this.

The tastes are also individually described on pages 42–8, but if you want to check a specific food, and whether it's a good food for your specific dosha, you should also check the Taste Table (pages 153–64).

It can sound tricky, but truly, it's not. Knowing the rasas that are best for you makes food selection very simple. If you can eat more *sweet* food, you know you're good with meat, dairy and grains. If you can eat more *pungent* food, you know you can enjoy spicier meals – so, more chilli, garlic, onion, etc. This becomes second nature very quickly, and is what makes the Ayurvedic way of eating practical and painless.

Being 'diagnosed' as Pitta–Kapha was the most fascinating point of my journey, because I realized I often ate the wrong sort of food. Despite thinking my choices were very healthy and ought to nourish me, I often felt 'wanting' after I'd eaten them. I love fruit, but I was eating a lot of citrus and grapes because they're regulars in those convenient ready-prepared supermarket fruit bowls you can grab on the go, and I never particularly enjoyed them. Learning about my dosha, I found out that I need to eat riper, sweeter fruits which don't tax the body, and that pears, cherries, strawberries and apricots were all great for my Pitta–Kapha personality. Funnily enough, they are among my very favourite fruits – I just hadn't gone out of my way to buy and eat them.

I'd been eating the wrong fruit because I thought any fruit was good enough, but if I'd actually listened to my appetite I would have chosen a juicy apple in the loose produce section instead. Lesson learned, and no more pre-prepared supermarket salads for me. Now I eat the fruit I fancy, fresh, seasonally and where possible locally too, which makes a really big difference to the nutritional value that is passed on to my body (learn much more about seasonality in Chapter 6).

When I started learning about the rasas, I made a mental list of all the meals I find most satisfying. Satisfying – by my definition and one that will play a crucial role in the Body Balance Diet – is food that you feel happy having eaten. It fills the gap, yes, but it also satiates on another level: it's hit the spot, satisfied all the cravings and needs within your body that perhaps you weren't even aware of in the first place. In my experience, the meals that satisfy me most do so because they offer a balanced and rich variety of tastes, or rasas, along with interesting textures to boot. By better understanding the rasas, you'll soon be able to cook in a way that puts the most complementary ingredients together, in a way that will really help your body thrive.

So, Which Tastes Are Good for You?

When we talk about the rasas we also talk about their effect on your dosha. Bringing your dosha into balance is at the crux of this diet, and at the heart of Ayurveda itself. We want to get to a place where all the five elements within us are optimal and settled and our body is therefore functioning at its best.

It's best to eat the rasas which are at the opposite end of the spectrum to your own dosha, and will thereby reduce it. For Pitta, that's Bitter (Air and Ether), Astringent (Earth and Air) and Sweet (Earth and Water). For Vata, that's Sweet, Sour (Earth and Fire) and Salty (Water and Fire). For Kapha, that's Pungent (Fire and Air), Astringent and Bitter.

The rasa cheat (and eat) sheet below shows which rasa is good for your dosha:

Rasa Cheatsheet

Taste (Rasa)	Vata	Pitta	Kapha
Sweet	More	More	Less
Sour	More	Less	Less
Salty	More	Less	Less
Pungent	Less	Less	More
Astringent	Less	More	More
Bitter	Less	More	More

Is it Bitter or Astringent?

Many Ayurvedic doctors choose to classify rasas in a way that is quite complex – a spice such as turmeric, for example, can be classified as Bitter, Pungent and Astringent, all at once, but such a classification can make it difficult to know how and when, and how much of it, to use.

In the end, in consultation with several leading Ayurvedic practitioners and after extensive trialling of my recipes to ensure they're still as effective as possible, I've decided to classify the foods under their primary rasa (and this is true of all the foods listed in the Taste Table on pages 153–64 too). Turmeric does possess three rasas, but its action is primarily a light, drying one – which is why it is primarily Bitter.

Why Do You Crave Certain Foods?

When our dosha is serially, and seriously, imbalanced, we don't feel great and we find that instead of craving the foods that do us good, we tend to crave precisely those foods which do us no favours at all. Think back to the vicious cycle I mentioned in Chapter 1. If you're balanced, your body is more in tune with what it needs – I crave seasonal soups and hot winter salads bursting with veg – the stuff that does my body the most good. If I'm run down, stressed and overly tired, I often crave salty and overly spicy food.

Vata types tend to undereat or lose their appetites completely when they're stressed, or grab raw, cold, dry foods (salads, crackers, fruit), which does not help their constitution. Vata types must always eat well – particularly at lunchtime, when their digestive fire is strongest; they can enjoy a three-course lunch without weight gain.

Kapha types have a sluggish metabolism and are prone to comfort-eating, reaching for Sweet and fatty foods most often of all the dosha types. Kapha types frequently have small appetites (slow hunger) and even slower digestion. Kapha types don't cope well with some protein: light poultry and fish is fine, but they really can struggle to digest richer meats, and they don't actually need them as their body type does far better on lighter protein, and shifts stubborn weight when eating a lighter, cleaner, steamed diet – think lightly stir-fried food (tofu is good), with meals rich in pulses, beans, lentils and metabolism-boosting spices.

Pitta types might seek spicy, Salty food, but need cooling and calming down – you require foods that will break down slowly, and complex carbohydrates (whole grains, pulses and beans, brown rice, root veg . . . see the Taste Table on pages 153–64 for more) are a Pitta type's best friend. Though you may often crave an intense salty or spicy hit of flavour – I know I do when I'm imbalanced! – your body thrives on simple, soothing flavour. Avoid vinegary, sharp, acidic, tomato-based meals. Meat is also very acidic, so if you're craving a burger, opt for chicken if you can, and limit the amount of red meat and egg yolks you consume (egg whites are fine).

Pitta types can get very irritable when hungry (I know that feeling well). In general, snacking is not in line with Ayurvedic wisdom, but if there's going to be a long gap (more than four hours), plan ahead and pack a dosha-supporting snack such as vegetable crudités (try with my hummus or one of my 'pestos'), oat, spelt or rye crackers, and vegetable juices. You can cope well with raw food, so fruit and veg are often great foods for you. Try to eat these in season, and organic if possible.

There is much scientific discussion about whether or not organic fruit and veg have more vitamins than food that is grown non-organically. One benefit is certain: they are grown without the chemical interference that can meddle with your body's own internal balance. Eating for the seasons is particularly important in Ayurveda because it means you're balancing Vata, Kapha and Pitta more effectively, as the food you eat at the right time of the year naturally attunes your body – a key Ayurvedic tenet.

The Six Tastes

Sweet

Earth and Water dominate this taste, which has the qualities of being oily, damp and also quite heavy. It's good for reducing Vata and Pitta, but really increases Kapha. Dairy, meat, grains, starchy vegetables, nuts, pulses and beans – these are all Sweet. That may surprise you – after all, we're used to thinking of sugar as being sweet, but these Earth and Water foods all have a pleasing richness to them, they're not overly savoury or sharp on the palate. Most fruit is also Sweet. We don't digest Sweet foods quickly, but they are very nourishing and will make up the staple part of most diets. This needs to be what we eat most of, because it gives us the energy to live. But for Kapha types, too much Sweet can imbalance us, because Kapha is already made up of Earth and Water, so we need to pull back on as much dairy and meat as possible and focus more on vegetables.

Sour

Sour is mainly Fire – think of your taste buds and the saliva they produce when eating sour food, and how it warms up your mouth – but there is also a bit of Earth in there too. Sour food is great for reducing Vata, but increases Kapha and really increases Pitta. Foods include most fermented foods (wine, beer, yogurt, fermented cheese, soy sauce), pickled or vinegary food, and citrus fruit. This is a taste which you'll generally eat little of as these foods do not tend to form the staple part of one's diet, but it is great for rebalancing an excess of Vata. Also Sour are tomatoes (I'd recommend caution here – see the box below).

Tomatoes

Much of the food we eat contains tomatoes that are less than lovely – think of the pale, soggy, flavourless ones you often get in shop-bought cheese-and-tomato sandwiches – and they're often the base of pasta sauces, pizza toppings, soups . . . but tomatoes are acidic (they tend to have a pH of around 4) and don't help Pitta or Kapha types. However, if you eat them when they're wonderfully ripe and actually in season (generally from July to October), their pH is closer to 5. Enjoy them fresh in a salad, or crushed onto a piece of bread with a drizzle of lovely oil. If cooking them, cook only ripe tomatoes and they'll retain their less acidic nature (making a big batch of in-season tomato paste that can then be the base of pasta sauces or soups is a good idea too).

Salty

In Ayurveda, Salty is a rather literal taste as there are not many salty foods that occur naturally. Salty refers to food flavoured with sea/rock salt, soy or seaweed. Element-wise, it is made up of Fire and Water. Small amounts help digestion and also calm the nervous system. It's good for reducing Vata, but increases both Pitta and Kapha. I've read widely on this matter and some Ayurvedic practitioners list naturally salty fish too. Obviously much of the food we eat is salty – though not naturally so – and in fact 75 per cent of our daily salt intake comes from food we do not add salt to. These are most processed foods, such as sandwiches, cereals, soups, cheese, processed meats, cookies, crisps/potato chips and bread (for more on 'good' versus 'bad' bread, see pages 126–8), which can have a surprising amount of salt in them, so one must take these foods into account too if trying to cut down on salt intake. The World Health Organization recommends no more than 5g of salt a day for adults.

I love hummus, anchovies, crisps/potato chips and corn chips, and I thought my snacks were healthy (better than a bar of chocolate, surely?). I scarcely ever added salt to my food because I'd always been wary of the high blood pressure that one side of my family has always been prone to. So, although my home cooking was low-salt (in cooking I occasionally used Himalayan pink crystal salt or organic sea salt), the ready food I snacked on was laden with it. But as a Pitta–Kapha, Salty foods aren't on my ideal list. I wasn't sleeping well and my skin was dry; I was constantly thirsty despite drinking plenty of water, but never felt 'hydrated'.

My Ayurvedic doctor in the Maldives pinpointed my salt overdose almost immediately. He could feel it in my skin and saw that it was aggravating my Fire – completely imbalancing Pitta.

I realized I'd been consuming far too much cheese, take-away soup, smoked salmon and those aforementioned salty snacks (which are, I suppose, relatively healthy, but their sodium content does add up). As soon as I cut right back on salt my thirst balanced out, I slept far better, and my skin began to glow again too. An excess of salt in the diet can cause our systems to become overly acidic – redness of the skin and a tendency to rashes are giveaways here – and, of course, it can also lead to high blood pressure, and ultimately serious heart problems.

Bitter

Bitter is a combination of Air and Ether, and the qualities are light, dry and cold. It really reduces Kapha and Pitta, but increases Vata. Bitter foods are naturally purifying, they help the body to cleanse itself, and kickstart digestion and weight loss.

Bitter foods are often quite potent and nutrient dense, and most should only be eaten in small quantities. Spice-wise, turmeric, coriander/cilantro leaves and seeds, and fenugreek are primarily Bitter, as are certain fruits such as grapefruit, olives and bitter melon (also called bitter gourd, bitter squash, balsam pear or wild cucumber – botanic name, *momordica charantia*). The latter, I'll admit, is not readily available in supermarkets (though I've seen it in organic supermarkets and the odd 'boutique' greengrocery) but plays a big role in traditional Ayurveda. Bitter melon tea is also widely available via the internet; a hugely popular tea in India, it is said to stabilize blood sugar levels and is popular in the treatment of diabetes.

Another common Bitter food is coffee (see box).

Coffee – Yes or No?

The Ayurvedic community has rather a lot to say about coffee. While myriad studies have shown that drinking several cups of coffee a day can lower one's risk of developing cancer, diabetes, Parkinson's and heart disease, the results of the studies were similar with both caffeinated and decaffeinated coffee. It's the high antioxidant content of the coffee bean itself that's doing the magic, not the buzz you get from the caffeine.

But (and there's always a but) we also know that coffee makes us produce stress hormones, including cortisol – which is why you often get that fluttery-chest 'fight or flight' high after a cup. It also makes the brain produce dopamine, and it's this hormone that that makes it strongly addictive.

The main purpose of the Body Balance Diet is to bring everything into balance, and to bring the body out of the over-active stressed tense

---

state which is often the upshot of modern life. For this reason, coffee is not going to help an imbalanced body.

Vata types – who are flighty and active enough as it is – would do better largely to avoid coffee, and replace it with antioxidant-rich teas, such as rooibos, although a cup here and there is just fine. Pitta types are already quite fiery and driven, so coffee could push them toward the more aggressive end of the spectrum. In this instance, I'd say avoid a coffee on an empty stomach, but if it's after a healthy meal, and provided it's not a triple shot, it won't push you over the edge. Kapha types are calmer and more lethargic by nature, so by all means go ahead and enjoy a cup of Joe every now and again is unlikely to tip you off balance.

Astringent

You can recognize an Astringent food from the effect it has on the palate – think of the saliva-provoking tannins you get in red wine and the way it makes the mouth pucker up. If you've ever eaten an unripe banana you'll know that sensation. Wine and unripe bananas aside, there's also broccoli, cauliflower, asparagus, artichoke, celery, sprouts and green beans. Many fruits are partially Astringent too – cranberries and pomegranates most of all, but also less ripe pears and apples. Chickpeas, lentils, buckwheat, yellow split peas and alfalfa are all Astringent too. Made up of Earth and Air, Astringent foods really help to cool and dry the system – hence that dryness in the mouth when you eat them. This is a great thing for the damp or overly fiery Kapha and Pitta types, but doesn't do Vata any favours.

Pungent

This taste is made up of Fire and Air – it's heating and drying, but also light. It's good for reducing Kapha, but increases both Pitta and Vata. Pungent foods help stoke one's digestive fire (agni) and also shift mucus (so they're good to eat if you're suffering with chesty, phlegmy or snotty illnesses).

Pungent foods also get things moving – not just through the gut, but also within the blood – boosting circulation and shifting cholesterol.

The hottest (as in foods with natural 'chilli' heat), are all Pungent – think garlic, ginger, raw onions, mustard seed (and mustard greens), rocket/arugula, horseradish, and chillies, of course. Chia seeds are Pungent too. Many spices are primarily Pungent, including allspice, basil, bay leaves, black pepper, caraway, cayenne, cinnamon, cloves, cumin, lemongrass, nutmeg, oregano, paprika, parsley, peppermint, rosemary, saffron, sage, star anise and thyme.

Remember: always eat more of the foods that reduce your dosha. This will help keep your system balanced.

I've said before that I am by no means an Ayurveda puritan, and many Ayurvedic recipe books rely on grain- and pulse-rich vegetarian food, which can seem quite alien to Western palates. While I adore a good vegetable, lentil or chickpea curry, I also like cheese and chicken, yogurt and lamb, fish and bread. So, when in Chapter 1 I said you need to remove the rules to remove the guilt, I meant it. That's why the Rasa Cheatsheet on page 39 uses the words *less* and *more*. I don't believe in never.

I want to be able to enjoy a great burger or tacos, scrambled eggs and salmon, a fresh tuna mayonnaise sandwich . . . That's why I've worked on a plan that incorporates all the essential elements of the six tastes, while also using good, wholesome, natural ingredients to ensure that, yes, you can have your burger and eat it – but let's just tweak and tailor it first, to ensure you're giving your body what it really needs.

My Dosha Type is Confusing Me!

What if you're Vata–Pitta and as Vata you can eat lots of Sour, but as Pitta you can't? It's all a balancing act – and you should always give the strongest emphasis to your main dosha – but if both doshas are on an equal footing (which is not uncommon), you can continue to eat these 'contradictory' tastes, but just don't make them a staple part of your diet. Focus instead on the rasas which balance both doshas: for Vata–Pitta, that's Sweet (dairy, meat, grains).

Build your meals around this food, but you can still dip into the good-for-Vata and good-for-Pitta flavours as and when you really want them (as you'll see from my recipes at the back of this book). If you're tri-doshic, the key thing for you is to eat seasonally, as imbalances are not very often caused by your constitution (which is inherently balanced), but rather by the environmental shifts we experience every year. You will need to eat foods that pacify Pitta in hot weather (late spring, summer); pacify Vata in cold, windy, dry weather (ordinarily autumn and spring); and pacify Kapha in wet, cold weather (winter).

four

OPTIMIZE YOUR DIGESTIVE POWER

There's a great word in Ayurveda which describes the power of your digestion – agni – literally, your digestive fire. It's all very well talking about balance and metabolism and eating seasonally and so on, but if your digestive system is seriously up the spout, not only will you be unable to absorb all the wonderful nutrients from the food you're eating (which will leave your system wanting), but you'll also find it difficult to shift stubborn excess weight.

If the Body Balance Diet is a new beginning for you, it must also follow that it will be a fresh start for your digestive system. The Body Balance Diet does away with so many ways of eating which stress, overload and dampen your digestion, and it steadily encourages your body to regain full digestive and metabolic strength, getting the very best from all the food you eat, every time you eat.

How do you know if your digestive fire is already good? Simple: you feel wonderful. Your eyes are bright and sparkling, your skin glows, your tummy is settled (rarely gassy or growly), you sleep well, you have very regular bowel movements and eat regular meals without cravings in between. Your agni is balanced.

There are three other types of agni:

- **Irregular** – your tummy is all over the place – you're frequently bloated, constipated and crampy and can suffer with gas, indigestion and hard, dry stools. Your appetite isn't regular either: some days you'll eat next to nothing, other days you'll be supremely hungry and eat lots of big meals. This erratic nervy energy is common in Vata types.

- **Weak** – you do not have a big, healthy appetite – instead, you are slow to hunger, but also slow to digest. You often feel heavy and lethargic after a meal and can go a long time without passing a stool. Your tummy often feels 'full' (a sign that your digestive system is backed up), and you often get intense cravings for very sweet food, tea and coffee. This digestive type is most common in Kapha.

- **Intense** – when you're hungry it is a very powerful feeling – it can come on suddenly and leave you feeling light-headed, desperate to find food as soon as possible! Intense thirst is common too; you often have dry lips and a dry mouth, even if you're drinking lots of water. Your stools are often loose, and you're more prone to heartburn and stomach acid than other doshas. This is true of Pitta types.

The goal of the Body Balance Diet is to restore every individual to their balanced digestive state: where you wake up clear-headed, go to bed calmly, go about your day brimming with energy and can honestly answer 'great' when people ask how you are feeling. We feel well, not only because our bodies are working optimally, but also because our minds are best-supported by a truly nourishing and nurturing diet. We naturally feel more optimistic when we eat well. Contrast that with the lazy, heavy feeling you get after having eaten a stodgy, fatty lunch or full fried breakfast. While you may feel wonderfully full at first, soon you'll simply want to curl up and go to sleep, and the thought of walking home fills you with dread: 'I can't move!' That's not natural and it's not healthy. We should feel revitalized by food, not (literally) weighed down by it.

Perhaps you've experienced that truly alive feeling on holiday, if you've left the daily grind and consequent junk food behind, and travelled somewhere where you ate only wonderful fresh seasonal nutrient-dense food for a week? Did you gain a spring in your step, a glow in your skin, a sparkle in your eye? Did people keep asking what you'd 'done', because you looked so well? That's the power of the right food. Food that can heal, beautify, strengthen and support us, inside and out – but, crucially, food that's also eaten when you're calm and relaxed, which makes ALL the difference.

How to Balance Your Digestion and Stoke Your Fire

First up, a struggling stomach will need a spring clean. I believe this can be done with some breaking of old habits and some sensible dietary changes. I do not subscribe to colonic irrigation myself as I believe that if you eat the right foods for your body, and foods that also ignite your digestive juices, there's no need to be 'cleared out'. You'll feel light and energized, naturally. Having said that, I've been in the industry long enough to know that there are good and bad colonic practitioners out there (and I do have friends who've been having regular colonics for years and swear by them), but I also feel there's some level of 'shock' involved in a colonic, because the process is unnatural, in that it's not something your body would ever do by itself. I know far too many people who've struggled to gain digestive balance afterwards – the flora of the gut being disturbed by the process.

Instead of colonics, I therefore endorse an Ayurvedic immersion diet, which will get the body to expel its waste naturally, and will also ensure that you're not messing around with the very complex flora of the gut. It's an ideal place to start because it will very gently ease you into a balanced state, and then help ensure that you remain there. I don't believe in doing anything overnight – I feel that any significant change takes time, and it ought to take time because that is what makes your body and mind receptive to it. You need to do an unfamiliar thing many times before it feels natural. I was reminded of this quite recently with my second child.

Despite breastfeeding being viewed as the most natural interaction there is – one assumes baby is born knowing how to suckle (although, very sadly, this is not always true), and that mother instinctively knows how to feed – it is, in fact, a process that often comes with a great deal of pain and angst. I struggled a great deal with my first child and almost gave up every day, until, at around three months of age, something clicked and it became 'natural'. That was after doing eight or more daily feeds, every couple of hours, for 12 weeks. I remind myself of this whenever I hope to quell a habit of mine or adopt a new lifestyle change. All change takes time. If you are committed to moving toward a more Ayurvedic way of life, this will take time too. It's relatively painless, but it does take time before it feels as if you were born to do it.

Alongside my immersion diet, I also extol the benefits of following the 10 simple steps below. They're small changes and you can make some or all of them, in the knowledge that every little helps your gut get a step closer to that 'balanced' feeling.

10 Steps to a Balanced Digestive System

1. Hot Wake-up Call

Before you do anything in the morning, boil your kettle and fill half a mug with boiling water, then the other half with room temperature filtered water. Drink as it is, or with a squeeze of lime if you're feeling bloated or constipated, or with grated ginger if you're feeling very lethargic. If your system is really backed up, try leaving a teaspoonful of linseed (also called flaxseed) soaking in a glass of warm water for 10 minutes, then drink it down, along with the seeds (best on an empty stomach, but can be taken throughout the day).

The feeling of warm water hitting the stomach first thing in the morning is quite incredible because it's pouring down a pipe that's not been used in hours. Try and leave at least 20 minutes before breakfast. It's the quickest and easiest perk- and pick-me-up there is.

2. Try Triphala

A traditional Ayurvedic remedy (available as a capsule-form supplement) for gentle gut cleansing, Triphala is made from three traditional Indian fruits (haritaki, amla and bibhtaki) and also contains psyllium, liquorice, fennel and linseed – gold-standard gut-clearers! The beauty of this supplement is that it need not be taken as part of a fast. Ideal in partnership with the Ayurvedic immersion, this will have the body humming before the week's end.

3. Get Spice Savvy

My Turkish Cypriot background may not be Ayurvedic, but we do know a thing or two about herbs and spices, and whenever I had an upset tummy as a child, my mother would boil up a generous pinch of fennel seeds in water (the water should boil up and turn a pretty yellow-green colour) and get me to drink it. Within minutes my stomach used to start to feel better. The drink is lovely and mild with a herbal aniseed-like flavour – not sharp or bitter as you might expect – and I now make it for my three-year-old whenever she's got what she calls a 'bubbly tummy'. Fennel is a truly great gut-calmer, as is ginger, which can be added to all foods or boiled up in hot drinks.

Another Turkish tea I make for relatives (we call it *kokulu çay* – fragrant tea) includes 8 to 10 cloves, one large broken-up piece of cinnamon bark and a large pinch of cumin and fennel seeds. Place these ingredients in a strainer and run boiling water over them to rinse away any sediment or dust, then use the spices in the strainer to make your tea, just as you'd use tea leaves. Or boil them up in a pan of whole goat's milk, add a bit of sugar, strain and drink. It makes a delicious creamy sweet masala chai, filled with spices that all support the cleansing and strengthening of the gut.

Other spices that are great to add to your diet when you're feeling off-colour are ginger, ground coriander, turmeric, cumin and black pepper – all of which are Ayurveda's secret weapons for stoking and restoring digestive fire.

4. It's Fruit O'Clock

I love fruit, particularly in the summer when I crave it like a crazed person. For years I used to eat a bowl of fruit after dinner and had actually reached the point where I thought I had irritable bowel syndrome (IBS) because I would always experience significant discomfort after large meals. Now I realize that there is a time and a way to eat fruit, and it isn't alongside or soon after any other food. Fruit is very easily digested – it contains some fibre, but is primarily fructose and breaks down quickly in the stomach. So, if you eat it after a meal and it lands on top of some complex carbohydrates or protein, you will end up with food that's being broken down by different enzymes, at different rates. The result? A lot of messy gut activity, and gas, as a byproduct. Hence my mistaken IBS assumption. My gut pains were not medical, they were simply down to having eaten fruit at the wrong time.

Ayurveda is very specific about fruit and suggests it is always best eaten on an empty stomach. So after your glass of warm water in the morning, enjoy ripe fruit at room temperature. This is how we were meant to eat it – sun-warmed, first thing, fresh from the tree.

When fruit is refrigerator-cold it shocks the stomach, which hinders optimal digestion. Almost all fruits taste better and sweeter at room temperature – particularly berries, peaches, apricots and melon. Get into the habit of taking fruit out of the refrigerator the night before and eating it about 40 minutes before breakfast.

Another good time to enjoy fruit is mid-morning, as a snack before lunch, as you want to try to leave a couple of hours on either side – so breakfast before 9am, fruit between 10 and 11am and lunch around 1pm won't tax those digestive juices. For more on what to eat, and with what, see Chapter 5.

5. Take Your Time

Some doshas really do need to take more time than others over their meals: Kapha with their sluggish digestion benefit from spending a longer time chewing; Pitta, with their tendency for internal fire, do well to eat quietly in a peaceful spot; and Vata types, who often suffer digestive upset and loose bowels, need to slow down the eating process completely, savour each mouthful, and never eat on the go (which is a common tendency with airy, and busy, Vata types).

6. Be a Probiotic Pro

Achieving optimal gut health (and digestive fire) is at the heart of Ayurveda. One of the simplest ways to aid digestive fire is to boost your stomach's healthy bacteria with a proven probiotic blend, particularly after a course of antibiotics or during illness. I am calling on modern wisdom here. Obviously ancient Ayurveda doesn't have a stance on probiotics – but I've found, from trial and error, that my digestive fire is always strongest when I support it with probiotics and enzymes (see Step 7 below). We often hear that our immune system is situated in our gut: what this means is that 70 per cent of the antibacterial and antiviral cells within our body are situated in the walls of the stomach and intestines. Our stomach also produces acid, which kills off most pathogens, and our small intestine produces mucus, which blocks further potential pathogens from entering our bloodstreams. So, when your gut lining is weakened, your immunity will also be compromised. I really cannot overstate the importance of a healthy stomach in the pursuit of good overall health! For this reason I recommend taking a proven daily probiotic (see Resources, page 220).

7. Eat Your Enzymes

Some doshas struggle with protein or carbohydrate digestion more than others, but all can benefit from a good comprehensive digestive enzyme. If we ate only natural nutrient-rich food, our digestive enzymes would do a fine job of extracting the nutrients we needed from them, thereby sufficiently fuelling our bodies. And if we were to eat solely raw fruit and raw vegetables (I wouldn't recommend it – see below), the enzymes we need to digest them are already contained in these foods, but these enzymes can be depleted if the soil the food is grown in is low in nutrients (and this is increasingly the case for environmental, climatic and economic reasons). For these reasons I feel it's best to err on the safe side (and digestive enzymes are deemed universally safe) and invest in a good digestive enzyme, which can be a real boon to all.

Interestingly, we also produce fewer gut enzymes as we get older (at age 50 around half as much as we do at age 20), so it's a sensible support mechanism as we age too. Look for a good combined enzyme (which will help with all food digestion, including fats, protein and carbohydrate) in capsule form. (See Resources, page 220.)

8. Guard Against Gas

Once you're eating better, following some of the guidelines above, and benefiting from digestive enzyme and probiotic support, you should start to feel a lot better. But should a rogue meal hit your stomach hard, and leave you with windy-pops (my daughter's words) I've found three things that help nicely:

1 the fennel tea I described earlier, sipped slowly after the offending meal;

2 a fresh mint tea; or

3 a chew on the simple and effective Conscious Food D'Mix, which is packed full of seeds and leaves that, when chewed for upward of a minute, then swallowed, do a great job at shifting that gas.

Incidentally, I tried all of the above very soon after having my second child, when gas is often a problem due to the weakening of the abdominal muscles during the strain of childbirth, and found this last one to be most effective, and far more so than chemist/drugstore alternatives.

9. To Snack, or Not to Snack?

First things first: you need to get better acquainted with your body. A lot of people leap toward the vending machine at the first sign of hunger, but it could simply be thirst, boredom or habit. Get used to the light feeling in your body when you've fully digested your previous meal, and your thoughts turn once more to what you might eat. Try to get away from eating insubstantial snacks all day long, which never satisfy, are never fully digested, and mean that you never stop thinking about food! If you're eating properly you shouldn't need to snack very often. If you start to feel hungry sooner than expected, drink a cup of herbal tea or warm water first. Sometimes it's thirst you're feeling. A good complex breakfast will satisfy for four hours, taking you from 8am to noon, lunchtime.

But if you're eating breakfast earlier and having lunch later, a snack may be necessary – do not let yourself get over-hungry or light-headed. Simply pack a snack from the many options listed at the back of this book, and enjoy it three to four hours after your previous meal, and two hours before you will have your next (this works if you're someone who breakfasts at 7am, snacks at 11am and lunches at 1pm). Swot up on delicious dosha-specific snacks at www.balanceplan.co.uk.

10. And Breathe . . .

I've talked about how vital it is to eat slowly and mindfully rather than as a means of filling up, as quickly as possible – then going about your day again. I know how tough it can be to find time to eat in a busy job (as an office 'junior' I was once told I could eat when my editor ate – which was *never*). I suppose it's a balancing act: if you do work in a place that supports your right to sit on a park bench and savour your sandwich, or in a quiet canteen sipping your soup, then please take advantage of it. If you don't, then try to ensure that, whenever mealtimes are your own – breakfast or dinner, perhaps – you savour them, you chew well, eat slowly, and stop your mind from racing onto the inevitable, 'once I've eaten this, I can get up and do X, Y and Z.' Eating keeps us alive, so we owe the process a bit of time, and respect.

five

WHAT GOES WITH WHAT, AND WHEN?

So, now you know how to stoke your digestive fire and have an idea of the sort of foods that do and don't work for your body type, the question is how to put this knowledge into action to ensure your body learns to process food easily and efficiently. There's another layer to Ayurveda, which sits hand in hand with the tastes that you should eat more of – it's the way certain foods ought, or ought not, to be combined.

Food combining is based on the idea that certain foods are more easily digested on their own, or with certain other foods. Other combinations are far less digestible, causing you to suffer stomach upset, heartburn and bloating. The concept of food combining is not exclusive to Ayurveda, but Ayurveda's combining guidelines do predate any others, and are rather different to some of the other combining 'rules' you may have read. It's not a matter of protein with protein and carbohydrate with carbohydrate (which I've always considered to be the most limiting stance of all!). No, Ayurvedic food combining is based on the foods that sit well together – according to their tastes, but also their effect on our bodies. If you combine, and eat according to your dosha, you will feel good after your meal – comfortable and energetic. This is the aim with every meal we eat, when we eat according to Ayurveda.

Is it Complicated?

One of the main complaints that people have about Ayurveda is its 'complexity'. So many foods are 'off limits', and even those that are fine cannot be eaten with certain other foods. I'm sympathetic to this, because I did have to make some changes to my diet and my mindset, but what was also true was that I needed to make them, because my diet was causing me to bloat, preventing me from dropping those extraneous pounds I'd gained from stress and a sedentary job, and balancing neither my digestive system nor my body as a whole. I didn't find the process complex so much as different: it took some getting used to, and I must have consulted the Combination Cheatsheet below 20-odd times a day at the beginning, but soon enough I learned that eating fruit with yogurt wasn't ideal, eating beans with fish was inadvisable, and that eggs are better eaten with grains than with fish or cheese. I would stress here, however, that if you've been eating something a certain way for many years and it's never been the cause of digestive upset, you are probably okay to continue eating it. I allow myself scrambled eggs and smoked salmon quite often – even though it breaks that egg and fish rule – because I feel great afterwards and enjoy every mouthful. But as soon as I cut out yogurt with fruit (I now add honey for sweetness to organic goat's or sheep's milk yogurt), I felt so much better and saw a significant reduction in my morning bloated belly. So, trust your instincts on this: as with every part of the diet plan, your intuition is your best friend in the pursuit of life-long body balance.

Combination Cheatsheet

Try not to eat . . .	with . . .
Eggs	beans, cheese, fish, fruit, milk, meat or yogurt
Fruit	any other food
Grains	fruit
Honey	boiling water
Hot drinks	cheese, fish, mango, meat, starchy carbohydrates or yogurt
Lemon	cucumber, milk, tomato or yogurt
Melon	any other fruit or any other food
Milk	most fruit (except dates) – banana and melon in particular – yeast-based bread, fish, rice dishes, meat or yogurt
Nightshade family: aubergine/ eggplant, potato, tomato, capsicum peppers	melon, cucumber, milk, cheese or yogurt
Beans or pulses	cheese, eggs, fish, fruit, milk, meat or yogurt
Yogurt	cheese, eggs, fish, fruit, milk, meat, nightshades or hot drinks
Large amounts of raw food	cooked food

Other Combining Considerations

We often think of yogurt as being a great healthy food, but the Ayurvedic jury's out on this one. I've found from experience that if I eat yogurt with a bit of honey in it, I am normally fine in the summer, but whenever I have a lot of yogurt in the winter, a snotty episode often follows in its wake. For this reason, I tend to avoid yogurt as soon as the weather turns, when I'm more prone to colds anyway.

Ayurvedically, foods with cold, wet and heavy qualities (such as yoghurt and ice cream) do not help our bodies. They weaken the digestive system, cause sluggishness (at best) and at worst, can even make us coldy, mucus-laden and congested. A large bowl of ice cream (sorry) is a pretty perfect culprit.

Ayurvedic puritans never combine milk with bananas, bread, fish or meat. The reasoning is that milk is a meal in itself and was designed that way (babies don't have breast-milk with a side of fries). Milk with certain grains, however, is fine – it's the cooking that helps here too, as with my porridges, which I've never had a problem digesting.

Be careful with honey and maple syrup. Many people add them to hot drinks to bring sweetness, but if you add either to boiling hot water, they become what Ayurveda deems 'toxic'. Heating them up essentially changes their properties, and makes them more glue-like once ingested. Ayurveda believes this causes it to stick to the membranes of the gut, where it festers and becomes noxious. Keep it below 40°C/104°F (so add once the water has cooled to drinkable temperature) and you'll be fine.

Ayurveda also suggests that we avoid eating raw and cold food with cooked, hot food. In moderation, you'll be okay – a simple side salad of leaves accompanying your dinner, for example, is fine - but if you're eating a big, mixed selection of raw vegetables with a hot stew or soup, you'll certainly be hindering agni. You digest cooked and raw food at different rates so you'll end up with digested mush and half-digested veg in your gut, which leads to gas and bloating. Wherever possible, you should try to eat all warm or hot food together (lightly steaming the vegetables you use in a chopped salad, for example, is an easy way to do this), and eat as little of that hard-to-digest raw food as possible – particularly if you're Vata.

Get the Juices Flowing

Eating foods with a sour, spicy or salty flavour literally gets our saliva flowing – and anything that does this will have a similar effect on the digestive juices. This is great, preparing the body for the incoming meal. Some fresh olives, nuts, lemony hummus or organic bread with a drizzle of chilli oil is a nice pre-dinner snack. Kapha types also benefit from eating Bitter appetizers – a green salad is just the ticket.

Regulate Your Mealtimes

The body finds balance more effectively when it's on a schedule (this is often true of much of our lives). Get used to meals at set times whenever possible, but accept that there will doubtless be times when this isn't possible. Make up for it with a nourishing, calming and entirely wholesome meal later that same day.

I see this with my children, who have breakfast, lunch and dinner at almost exactly the same times every day; it has really stoked their appetites and kept their digestions strong. But if we're out for lunch and things don't go to plan, I try not to fret – we simply return home, I let the girls work up good appetites again, and then we'll sit down to a better dinner to right the wrongs of the rushed/unhealthy/insubstantial lunch.

The Spice Passport

You can use certain spices with certain foods in order to boost their digestibility. I call this the spice 'passport', because it gives you a holiday from food-combining hassle! Cooking with ginger, clove, fennel, black pepper, cumin and cinnamon can really help us digest our food. Great for stews, soups and curries, mix and match your spice combinations until you find something you really like, in the knowledge that you're helping your body eat foods that might otherwise be difficult to digest.

I remember my Ayurvedic doctor in the Maldives talking to me about the benefit of cooking in a pot. By stewing something, or making several ingredients into a cohesive soup, for example, the process of cooking different ingredients together over a period of time can cancel out the constituent foods' inherent issues. Perhaps because the food is left to cook down to a point when it's more easily digested by the stomach, or because of the way in which the foods meld into one another, it is a great way to eat meat and grain together and why I've dedicated a small section to One-Pot Wonders at the back of the book.

Now that you've learned which tastes are best for your dosha, and which combinations are best for us all, there's another lovely, simple statement that applies universally to all of us, wherever we are, whatever we do. It is the central tenet of Ayurvedic eating:

Try to eat simpler meals.

That's it!

One can't argue with the fact that when presented with a huge burger, with its bread bun, cheese and pickles and tomato, and fries or onion rings on one side, a shake or soft drink on the other, the stomach is going to struggle. It's just the way it is. If I am going to eat something like that, I will definitely be taking my digestive enzymes before that meal! The simpler our meals, the less artificial, the fresher – the easier they are to digest.

six

HOW TO FIND BALANCE, ALL YEAR ROUND

This chapter is at the heart of the book for a reason – it is designed to nurture and support you and give you information that you can draw on for the rest of your life. Ayurveda is the foundation upon which I have built my life – the way I eat and the way in which I seek to balance my frenetic modern lifestyle – but I also have other tools in my wellbeing toolbox which I call upon year after year. Seasonality is a crucial part of understanding and maintaining body balance. It is a key tenet of Ayurveda too, one which we have grown further away from as our lives become increasingly urban, and we become removed from the subtle shifts within, and between, the seasons

Throughout the Body Balance Diet Plan I stick to the belief systems that support our modern way of life and that are also supported by both modern science and common sense. I've focused on traditional, but simple Ayurvedic advice that really helps weight-loss while boosting wellbeing. I have many friends who work in the Ayurvedic fields and whom I have consulted in the writing of this book, and I respect them because they very much live in this 'real world'. They are also, like me, naturally cynical and opposed to 'new age' schools of thought, and the things they prescribe and subscribe to are the things they themselves have tried, tested and chosen to trust. This is true of me too and the recipes and plans you'll find as you read on.

In this chapter, I explore the crucial importance of seasonality. I've already touched on this topic several times, but here I'll be providing a comprehensive look at how adopting a seasonal diet can naturally and simply transform your health. I've consulted leading seasonality expert, Annee de Mamiel, who runs a thriving acupuncture and traditional Chinese-medicine-based clinic in London, as well as producing two exquisite holistic beauty ranges. Her knowledge of how to shift our lives in line with the seasons is truly insightful, and since I've started living according to her advice, I've felt stronger, calmer, happier, and – yes – more balanced.

The Seasonal Secret of a Balanced Body

Long before seasonality was lauded by top chefs and nutritionists, Ayurveda extolled the virtues of eating as close to nature, and following its rhythm, as much as possible. Of course, eating seasonally was a way of life 5,000 years ago – you ate what nature produced for you, as you had no means to survive otherwise! But Ayurveda understood that we feel differently from season to season, that our bodies and minds react one way to summer's heat and brightness, and react another way to winter's bitter cold. We are more prone to certain illnesses or discomforts at different times of the year; we crave different foods; we may sleep or dream differently. These seasonal changes are profound and they affect our dosha too. Not living in tune with the seasons can imbalance us, just as not eating seasonally can. Because Ayurveda is the science of life, its principles adapt and react to life's seasonal cycles, always. We have an inherent doshic constitution, as mentioned before – our prakruti – but quite naturally and predictably, our bodies also change throughout the 12 months of the year, in response to the changing world around us. I am Pitta, but in winter, my minority dosha, Kapha, always increases. The wet, damp, cold qualities of winter cause Kapha to rise, and so I begin to eat more foods to reduce Kapha, while also taking care not to aggravate Pitta too much.

Considering our own dosha, and the foods that help our constitution thrive, is the foundation, but considering how our dosha is affected by winter and spring, summer and autumn, is the bricks and mortar that rest upon the our doshic foundation. This allows us to take a truly responsive approach to our daily diet, based upon what we need from season to season. This is as intuitive and intelligent as wellbeing gets, yet it is so easy to do. You simply eat the foods that are right for your dosha and for the season. Eating seasonally is 'natural' – literally – nature produces what we need, when we most need it: 'stick to your ribs' root vegetables in winter when we require extra sustenance; water-rich melons in summer when we're susceptible to dehydration.

The more I researched Ayurveda, and the more nutrition experts I talked to, the more I realized that optimal health is just not possible if you do not eat in a seasonal way. Everything that Ayurveda is built on is about 'nature' – our own natural unchanging dosha type, our constitution, our true self – and so it follows that if we want to nourish ourselves in the most natural way we can, direct from nature, mucking around with our food as little as possible, we have to honour the seasonal rules.

We must also respect these rules because seasonality defines the way in which we live Ayurvedically. Ayurveda believes that the seasons are characterized by the three doshas.

Which Dosha for which Season?

Summer, being hot and bright, is naturally Pitta.
Autumn, being cold, blustery and often dry, is Vata.
Winter, with its inherent heaviness – dark, cold, wet – is Kapha.
Spring is primarily Kapha (but it's more complex than that – see below).

Ayurveda understands that the season is not simply the date. A cold, blustery, icy May day possesses the qualities of cold early spring, or even winter, not the onset of summer. Modern Ayurveda experts also note that these guidelines were built around a hotter climate and way of life. But, to a large extent, we do tend to share a basic idea of 'season' all over the world. Even if December in Oz is scorching, and freezing in New York, we still have our summers and winters, springs and autumns.

If you're living somewhere with very little fluctuation in the weather, you should live according to whatever season predominates (all those sunshine days in California, for example, make it perpetually Pitta).

Spring is fascinating and Ayurveda calls it the 'king of the seasons'. This damp, bright, blooming time brings us out of winter, so Ayurveda applies much of the same rules to the two seasons. It is primarily Kapha – we are coming out of hibernation and must do so gently. It is time for rebirth, to energize, to revive and start afresh. This is why I advise those buying this book to wait until spring before embarking upon the immersion diet. You really can do it at any time of year due to its gentle nature, but in spring we're more likely to have the mental resolve to support our bodily changes, and are therefore more likely to succeed with our long-term plans.

Ayurveda believes that if we adapt our lives to the seasons we will avoid the inevitable maladies that come when we're out of sync with the world around us. So we should anticipate what the weather will do. For example, when it shifts from early to late spring – going from brisk to warm – we can start to reduce the amount of heat-producing foods in our diet, to get our Pitta in balance, which will give us a head start when summer rolls around.

Likewise, trying to stop the body drying out at the end of summer (so, taking the Vata-reducing route), will give you the advantage in autumn when your lungs and skin might become dry (skin conditions such as eczema and dermatitis and dry coughs are common autumnal complaints). For many of us this is an entirely new way of looking at the world, but one with centuries of practice to support it.

What if Seasonal Eating is at Odds with My Dosha?

Ayurveda can at times seem to contradict itself. There's a very clear way of seasonal eating that is recommended by all Ayurvedic practitioners, but that can sometimes appear to fight your own doshic preferences. You're often told to reduce Kapha in winter by focusing on eating Bitter and Astringent foods, but if you are naturally of a Vata constitution, you stand to raise Vata greatly by eating these foods alone.

Though on first glance it can seem that Ayurveda has suffered a case of over-simplification, the converse is actually true. The reality of life, and the balance of our doshas season by season, is very complex. We are all made up of all three doshas and this balance is always in flux – affected by diet, of course, but also the seasons. So, our approach to balancing our body must take both seasonality and our own dosha type into account.

Within this chapter you'll find guidance for each season, but I've also ensured that the recipes at the back of the book also specify which is good for which dosha, and which season to eat it in too. This should remove any potential contradictions – an issue I'll admit I've had with almost every Ayurvedic book I've consulted while writing this one.

We must respond to the season's changes within our bodies and look to prevent their effects before they produce an imbalance, which is far harder to treat. We can only do this by eating differently in each and every season, but in a way that is still honouring our own dosha.

At Annee de Mamiel's perpetually booked-up London clinic, she performs a wonderfully intuitive Seasonal Attunement treatment. The focus is on balancing the body's energy meridians or chakras, and getting the body to a point where it can expel the previous season's literal and metaphysical waste, and move on, stronger and far more balanced, to the season ahead. For this reason, her seasonal wisdom, which draws upon nutrition, Chinese medicine, acupuncture, breath work and aromatherapy, is truly integrative and produces the sort of results which have given her a year-long waiting list.

My Three Seasonal Health Secrets

Annee de Mamiel

1. Always Choose Seasonal Nutrition

Plants get their nourishment from the sun and soil. Seasonal fresh produce has been allowed to ripen in the environment it has evolved for and so it has optimal flavour and appeal – it's crispy, fragrant, juicy and colourful. The plant has also had the sun exposure it needs, which means it will have higher levels of antioxidants. The natural cycle supports seasonal produce and is perfectly designed to support our health too. Apples grow in the autumn and they are the perfect transitional food, helping the body get rid of excess heat and waste before winter.

In the spring the abundance of leafy greens helps us alkalize our systems and detox after a long winter of heavier foods. Our Western guts – fuelled by sugar, wheat and dairy (all acidic foods) – are often very acidic themselves. In the summer we need to cool down and stay hydrated by eating more fruit, berries, cucumber and watermelon. Building a lifestyle around seasonal food facilitates the body's natural healing process, and embracing the natural rhythm of things also helps simplify our lives by reducing our options. While you may be able to buy melons all year round now, it doesn't mean you should! As far as possible, stick to what has just been grown and harvested in the climate you are in, and harvest the healing energy of nature every time you do so.

2. Enhance Your Wellbeing with Essential Oils

Essential oils are a powerful way to improve our emotions as they act directly on our limbic system, affecting our physiological responses and how we feel. If we choose oils that have an affinity with the season, the benefits will be greatly heightened.

- **Spring** – look for oils that link to woody notes, to help reduce stress and irritability, and ease your frustration and anger. Try lavender, bergamot, peppermint, chamomile (Roman and German), grapefruit and ylang ylang.

- **Summer** – choose light, energizing and cooling herbaceous oils that will soothe the heart and promote peace of mind, love and joy within you. Try jasmine, melissa, neroli, palmarosa, rosemary, rose, ylang ylang and lavender.

- **Late Summer** – focus on healing to promote care, support and sympathy within you, helping you to think clearly and feel nurtured and supported, while grounding you and returning you to your centre. Try lemon, grapefruit, thyme, marjoram and vetiver.

- **Autumn** – use oils which will strengthen and support the lungs and boost the immune system, while also encouraging the breath and helping us to release and let go of anything that no longer benefits us. Try eucalyptus, cypress, fragonia and elemi.

- **Winter** – this is the time to strengthen your inner core, rest and replenish. It's also the time to release fears and fortify yourself so you have a platform of energy for the New Year. Try geranium, juniper, cedarwood, cypress, ginger and vetiver.

3. Breathe Right

Breath is life! It is the flow of energy. Survival without it is measured in minutes. Breathing is so important that you do it without thinking. Your breathing is the voice of your spirit. Its depth, smoothness, sound and rate reflect your mood. If you become aware of your breath and breathe the way you do when you are calm you will become calm. Practising regular, mindful breathing can be *both* relaxing and energizing.

Focusing on the breath is one of the most common and fundamental techniques for accessing a meditative state. Breath is a deep rhythm of the body that connects us intimately with the world around us.

Simple Breathing Exercise

Close your eyes, breathe deeply and regularly, and observe your breath as it flows in and out of your body. Give your full attention to the breath as it comes in, and your full attention to the breath as it goes out. Whenever you find your attention wandering away from your breath, gently pull it back to the rising and falling of the breath.

Inhale through your nose slowly and deeply, feeling the lower chest and abdomen inflate like a balloon. Hold for five seconds. Exhale deeply, deflating the lower chest and abdomen like a balloon. Hold for five seconds. Do this three or four times, then allow your breathing to return to a normal rhythm.

You will begin to feel a change come over your entire body. Gradually you will become less aware of your breathing, but not captured in your stream of thoughts. Your focus will become more inward. You will just 'be there'.

Keeping Your Balance through the Seasons

How to Thrive in Spring

We're coming out of winter, a time when Kapha is at its highest – think of the dampness we carry in our systems if still throwing off chesty coughs and colds, and also the lethargy we're left with after months of darkness.

Spring naturally supports change, and Ayurveda places a lot of store in this season, when it's all about getting rid of the Kapha that's built up within our bodies. We hear a lot about 'fresh starts', and perhaps the term has become hackneyed, but I'll never forget the year when I returned from a 10-day April escape (having left the UK after five solid months of rain, snow and far-lower-than-average temperatures) to find my garden blooming. My camellia tree was glorious – bursting with fat pink blooms, and all the little wildflowers along the garden path had sprung up, seemingly overnight. I have that picture emblazoned in my mind because it came with a huge accompanying sigh of relief. Feeling the spring sunshine on my face, looking up at that blue sky, taking a first full deep breath of warm air into my lungs, I knew that winter was over, I'd left repeated bouts of illness behind me, and now I could start to heal and move forward in both body and mind. Of course spring is not without its typical ailments: whenever flowers start to bloom, hay fever rears its head too, and Kapha types tend to suffer most. We're also in the process of getting rid of all that stagnant Kapha energy within our systems; the token spring cold is a symbol of that – and the body's own bid to spring clean itself.

By eating Ayurvedically and always in line with the seasons, you can really bolster your body against most health complaints, but you need to reset your way of life first. The easiest way to do this is to get your body clock back on track and in spring, we all benefit from waking along with the sunrise – before 7am.

Early waking dispels sluggishness, which is the cornerstone of Kapha. Kickstart your digestion and sharpen your mind. In lieu of hot water you can also try a cup of fresh, stimulating tea – grate ginger into boiling water, allow to cool and add a small drizzle of honey to taste.

Food-wise you should focus on Bitter, Pungent and Astringent flavours. These foods are naturally cleansing, and that's what spring is all about. Focus on light and fresh meals that are easy to digest – we don't want to add more stodge to a stomach that's in the process of shifting winter's excess. Food should, however, be warm – steamed, poached and grilled/broiled food is all great in spring.

Spicing is important – ginger, and most peppers (black, cayenne, chilli) are all good, but Pitta types be wary of overdoing it – we all need to shift the Kapha energy in spring, but we don't want to aggravate our doshas while we do it.

How to Thrive in Summer

Early summer takes us from spring's end up to summer solstice. Late summer leads up to the onset of autumn, and is when the scorching, driest days fall – it begins at a point when Pitta is at its highest and during this time Vata is also increased (the dry heat, as opposed to monsoon-like, humid weather, sparks Vata within us). Ayurvedic advice focuses on cooling Pitta down to prevent ourselves getting irritable, aggravated and unwell. Though many of us feel naturally healthier and more vital in summer, Pitta types are especially prone to getting flustered, and suffering the consequent heat and skin rashes and stomach upsets.

Get things on track by waking with the sunshine. Unlike in spring you needn't get up at sunrise, but listen to your body and try to wake yourself at a time when you feel most energized, which should be between 6.30 and 7.30am. If you have the opportunity for a short daytime nap (which would be blissful), sleep with windows open, in a light warm room, and if you know you'll be getting a good period of restful sleep at night, you can then fall into bed later in the summer without upsetting your body's balance – 11pm up to midnight is fine.

In summer, we can eat more salads than at any other time without it taxing our digestive system (as you know, I'm not a fan of all-raw all the time). It's best to eat them at lunchtime, though, and to make them up of the vegetables that best support your dosha. Too much raw food at night can imbalance Vata.

Look for Sweet, Bitter and Astringent flavours, which are naturally lighter and easier to digest. Naturally water-rich, sweet and cooling foods – particularly coconut – are wonderful at cooling the internal fire of the body. Mild coconut-spiced curries with basmati rice are excellent. Consuming your water via your food will help hydrate you on a far deeper cellular level than simply drinking gallons of water from a bottle (when it will often pass through your system without being adequately processed). Likewise, hydrating nut and grain milks such as almond and rice balance Pitta well and also offer supplementary minerals and vitamins. Adding a squeeze of lime to your water is another great way of cooling Pitta in the summer, as well as helping the body rehydrate faster.

In terms of alcohol, a beer is fine, as is wine, cider and vodka. But rum, brandy, whisky and red wine are all notoriously heating, and best forgone until autumn comes around again. In general, eating light and easily digestible foods is most important. Fruits and vegetables are at their greatest nutritional peak, giving us an abundance of choices that support healthy eating. It is particularly important to avoid overeating, especially as the summer gets later.

Foods that are cooling in nature are what the body craves, but don't have ice-cold drinks. If they are too cold, although the initial relief is pleasant, your system will get a shock – eating too much cold or raw food can actually injure the spleen and stomach, cause headaches, upset digestion and slow metabolism. Stick to room temperature if you can. Too hot won't help matters either, so tea and coffee drinkers, give your beverage a chance to cool, drinking it when it is warm rather than hot.

Meat-eaters should look for lighter flesh – in both colour and flavour – so chicken and both white and oily fish are best in summer. Red meat will very quickly imbalance Pitta further. It's also best to avoid citrus fruits – partly because they aggravate Pitta, but also because they're not summer fruits (they're harvested in late autumn and winter). Also avoid having too much tomato, chilli, onion and garlic, all of which will raise Pitta.

Aloe vera, as a morning drink before food, is recommended in summer as it both calms the stomach and helps cool the entire system. Similarly, teas made with rose, fennel and peppermint will help soothe you, and reduce Pitta.

How to Thrive in Autumn

With Vata on the up at the end of summer as the days become drier and cooler, the focus this season is on reducing Vata, and keeping the system warm, moist and hydrated, and one's mind calm.

Foods that support this are Sweet, Sour and Salty. Comfort is key at this time of year. As autumn becomes colder and wetter, we must once again focus on balancing Kapha.

Avoid eating too many cold and raw foods, which create dampness (upping our mucus and phlegm production). Grains are great: they are warming but also cleansing and so help with shifting Kapha at autumn's end too. Stock up on quinoa, barley and basmati rice and use as the base for many of your autumn meals.

Eat your vegetables warm and soft – steam for best results – and start enjoying seasonal soups and warming, silken stews again. Focus on foods that will ground you, dispelling that extra Vata and making you feel toasty and happy inside. Porridge is a great morning meal; when I was pregnant for the second time (and feeling both poorly and nauseous) my panacea was a cockle-warming Cardamom Chia Spice Porridge (see recipe on pages 173–4). Flavoured with maple syrup – another wonderful natural Vata-ridding food – this porridge is sweet, creamy, dreamy stuff, and chock-full of immunity-boosting antioxidants too.

Learn to enjoy and accept autumn's beauty. We're often sad to see the end of summer, but the stillness we can experience in autumn is unparalleled. It's a wonderful time to add an evening walk to your routine: wrap yourself and the family up warmly in layers of cotton and wool and head out to a quiet spot, taking in the changes around you – red, yellow and orange are all Vata-pacifying colours, so you'll be surrounded by a dosha-balancing canopy on every stroll. How lovely! Return to a cup of warm milk, spiced with ginger, cinnamon, nutmeg or cardamom (or mix them to taste), and then off to bed before 10pm, as we need more sleep to keep us fit, balanced and healthy once the sun starts setting earlier.

How to Thrive in Winter

For most of us, winter is cold, damp and cloudy – consequently, things can feel a bit sluggish. We move more slowly, we wake less eagerly, and many of us wander around harbouring a cough or cold and don't have that same 'zip' in our steps. This is all attributable to Kapha. At times, however, we can also experience Vata – on those bright, clear, icy-chill days – so if you have a Vata constitution, you must take care to keep Kapha at bay, while also pacifying your Vata.

As Kapha and Vata are at opposing ends of the dosha spectrum, whatever you eat to reduce Kapha will raise Vata. Therefore try to eat at least some foods that encourage Pitta. Look for ingredients with delicate natural spice, sweetness and also a satisfying, nourishing quality, without being too sticky, heavy or wet. Think of healthy, filling foods that are not processed 'stodge'. Filling foods can be well digested when you focus on wheat-free grains such as spelt, barley or quinoa – eaten with stews and soups. But also add more grain-rich meals in general to your diet – porridge, polenta and risotto (made with brown rice, barley or spelt is a great option) – and seasonal root vegetables, and also add more milk to the diet. If you can't tolerate lactose, then warming nut or grain milks, spiced with cinnamon, vanilla or nutmeg are the perfect thing to drink before bed.

Coming at the end of the year's cycle, it's normal for us to slow down during winter, and this is no bad thing. Our minds can be worn out, our bodies ready to hibernate – think of that urge we feel to settle down on the sofa and eat a hearty supper – this is all natural. What we don't want to do is succumb to complete lethargy and overeating, as that does not do the mood, or body, any favours. Though Ayurveda believes napping in both summer and autumn does you some good, it's not recommended in winter as it's far harder to shake off that sleepy malaise on darker days, and you'll end up carrying that heaviness around with you all day – which really raises Kapha.

The good news is, however, that we really can eat more in winter. Our digestive fire is always strongest in winter simply because we're designed to need that extra fuel. Most people's appetites tend to grow in the colder months and recede again once summer kicks in. This heightened digestive fire therefore makes winter the ideal time to enjoy some red meat once in a while, and all lean meats, particularly turkey and chicken, are fine too.

This is also the time of year to use more ghee – a type of clarified butter which is used extensively in Ayurvedic cooking. Because of my Mediterranean heritage, I use a great deal of olive oil in my cooking, and you'll see it in lots of my recipes. I know that it's good for you and I also think it tastes better than other alternatives.

I also use sesame, rapeseed/canola and coconut oils, which have their important and particular places. But there are certain recipes where only ghee will do, and in winter, when making certain rice, lentil or bean stews and soups, ghee is an important ingredient.

One would imagine that clarified butter is not particularly healthy, but ghee is the perfect transporter for both herbs and spices, ensuring that they are optimally absorbed and digested by the body. Ayurvedic doctors praise ghee's ability to nourish and 'oil' the body's connective tissues, muscles and joints, while also stoking your agni. It is therefore a great thing to keep in your store cupboard in winter (due to its purity, it does not require refrigeration). I would not, however, recommend lots of ghee to anyone with high cholesterol. Because I've tried continually to balance modern knowledge with the most salient Ayurvedic wisdom, I have used ghee in a recipe when only the unique properties of ghee will do, but I've used less-rich oils and fats in most other places.

Seasonal Attunement Treatment

There is a treatment called *panchakarma*, which is a godsend if you're the type of person who struggles through winter with cold after cold (a sure sign that Kapha is raging within you). If you can locate a good Ayurvedic clinic, or a mobile practitioner, this treatment will really get you on the right footing and will be performed at the end of autumn to give you and your immune system a headstart. It involves some serious gut-cleansing, which can feel unfamiliar (enemas are sometimes involved) – but is nevertheless far more gentle than colonic irrigation.

The process ordinarily involves three steps: *oleation*, which is the ingestion of seeds and oils to loosen and rid the body of internal blockages, toxins and waste, supported by massage; *bastis*, which are uniquely gentle and beneficial enemas, using special medicated herbal preparations; and *rasayana*, which is about restoring nourishment to your system once it has been cleansed, when it is at its most receptive.

The Western world tends to wait until January to 'detox' and attempt to lose weight (often via spartan and restrictive crash diets!) – but Ayurveda believes in a gentle, constant process of purification, supported by the seasons, and the body's own internal functions. To boost this natural process here are five simple but effective ways to boost inner cleansing and aid the loss of excessive weight. These principles work wonderfully all year round.

1. Satiate Hunger with a Glass of Warm Water, Honey and Lime Juice

Purifying and satisfying, when taken in place of a 'snack' this drink will often cancel out all hunger, and is therefore a great in-between-meals drink. Of course, if you do drink and enjoy it, but are still ravenous afterwards, then please, do eat! You can adjust the mix to taste, but a teaspoon of honey and teaspoon of lime juice in a large mug of warm water is about right.

2. Reinvent the Salad

I grew up in a house where we ate salad almost every day – not the sort of insipid, undressed side salad you often find in a restaurant, but a varied, bright, fresh, beautifully dressed, chopped salad that was always served with hot meals. Since becoming attuned to Ayurveda I've adapted my salads somewhat – I won't eat a completely raw cold salad with a big hot cooked meal – but because I still crave my salad fix with my dinner or lunch, I will lightly roast, steam or stir-fry the vegetables for my salad (from asparagus to capsicum peppers), so that they're warm and not wholly raw, and then make the salad up as normal. I take a lot of my salad inspiration from my Turkish culture. I just try to stick with the freshest seasonal vegetables, and dress them simply with virgin olive oil, lime juice and salt. I've also shifted the salad that I used to eat with my cooked food to the beginning of my meal, as a starter, and find it ignites agni – gets the digestive juices flowing – and means I eat a lighter main as a result. Ayurvedically speaking, it's a no-brainer – you're adding more Bitter and Astringent foods to a meal, which always helps shift Kapha (and excess weight), and said food is negligible in terms of fat and calories. I'd try to use lime more often than lemon, though, simply because according to Ayurvedic food principles lemon doesn't combine well with cucumbers or tomatoes – and both are mainstays of a regular salad.

3. Warm up Your Water – and Never Shock the Body with Cold Drinks

Ayurveda is very clear about this, realizing that cold slows the metabolism and hinders the stomach. As a wellbeing journalist I have often heard 'diet experts' recommend only drinking iced drinks, because it forces the body to burn off more calories in a bid to warm the water up to body temperature. Please don't listen to this! The calorie expenditure from this process is tiny and very unlikely to result in actual visible weight loss. What it will do, however, is cause an imbalanced, unhappy (and probably rather cold) internal body. Far better to stick to drinking warm water, which helps clear the colon, is far more effective in actually hydrating the body and respects the body's own internal environment, which can only ever be a good thing.

4. Swap Dinner and Lunch

If you are determined to lose weight, and can only make one change to your routine, it ought to be this. Eating a filling, healthy meal at lunchtime (with two or more courses) is the way to go. Lunch hits your stomach at a time when it's most receptive; the meal is better digested and boosts metabolism for the rest of the day, and is less likely to be eaten in a blind starving panic, which is what so often happens at dinnertime, when many of us ravenously raid the kitchen. In an ideal world, we'd eat lunch at noon and dinner at 5pm, but most of us are still sitting at desks at that time. If, therefore, you often leave six to seven hours between lunch and dinner, I always recommend a small snack around 4 or 5pm. This stops hunger spiralling into 'grab it and stuff it into my mouth' territory, and will then allow you to eat a lighter dinner, because the edge has been taken off your hunger. A small dinner, however, really requires a shift in psychology. We're used to sitting down at the end of a 'hard day', with a glass of wine and a big plate of food. It's a reward for making it through the day, but also our cue to switch off and begin eating, quite mindlessly, for much of the evening. If you can get yourself used to a big, lovely lunch instead, and the healthy late afternoon snack which is your 'appetizer', then your main meal once you're home ought to be nothing more complex than one of the many filling but 'lighter' dinners I've provided at the back of this book. It takes time to break years and years of habit, but once you get used to not feeling heavy at the end of the day, eating a smaller dinner earlier, and going to bed with a comfortable stomach, you'll come to love it.

5. Feed Yourself (Properly)

Okay, so I'm entering self-help territory here, but I'm afraid that food is an emotional subject; indeed, 'emotional eating' is now a recognized term (and one we've written about a lot at my magazine, *Psychologies*).

The truth is, if you're eating for myriad reasons that have nothing whatsoever to do with hunger, then this entire process

seven

A BALANCED MIND

Much of this book is focused on improving our mood – and good food certainly has the ability to do this – but there's also our psychology to consider – our default mental state, which is also at play within Ayurveda. Just as there are three doshas, which relate to the body, there are also the three main *gunas* (or *maha gunas*), which relate solely to the mind (Ayurveda leaves no stone, organ, thought or inclination unturned). The three gunas must be in balance if the mind is to be balanced, in just the same way that we endeavour to balance our three doshic elements, in order for us to achieve optimal physical health. As one might expect, the gunas can also be balanced through food, and each guna is related to a particular set of tastes or food types. This concept is yet another reason to love Ayurveda, highlighting how incredibly sage, forward-thinking and holistic this ancient discipline is. There are still doctors in the West who believe that food has little to no effect on our mental health – wholly denying any link between diet and depression. Depression is a complex illness with many aspects and triggers, but the foremost thinkers on mental health advocate a 'healthy mind' diet too – low in processed and refined foods, sugar, wheat, animal products . . . incredibly, the same stance taken by Ayurveda before the advent of Western medicine.

Ayurveda proffers the sane and sensible notion that what we eat makes us feel a certain way. (If you want to explore this idea, take a look at Further Reading and Resources on pages 217–20). Because gunas essentially relate to emotion and feeling, there are many, many more than the three main ones we touch on in this chapter – there are 20 that are commonly used and talked about, including eight that a lot of Ayurvedic experts refer to in terms of their relation to food, and subsequent feeling.

The Three Maha Gunas

Sattva – essence, purity, intelligence; creates balance

Rajas – activity and energy; creates imbalances

Tamas – substance; creates inertia

When we feel balanced, calm and happy, that is *sattva*. It is enlightenment: we are in harmony and at peace. We also feel loved and able to love – connected to the universe, stable and content.

Rajas is the force of change. It can make us feel energized and happy if it is short-lived, but eventually, the power of this passion leads to unhappiness, anxiety, conflict and distress. It is always upsetting the balance and fragmenting the whole.

Tamas is like the full force of gravity, keeping things pinned down, unable to move, inert, heavy and obstructed. It is characterized by a downward spiral – sinking deeper into decay, denial, sleep, shutting the world out and being unaware of anything else.

The three gunas also relate to three types of food. Each type of food brings about the effect that relates to that particular maha guna.

These gunas relate to many qualities, states, attributes, tastes . . . think of them as adjectives that can be used to describe a whole host of people, places and personalities.

- **'Sattvic' people** are healthy, creative, soulful and content. They are this way because they possess an adaptable and harmonious personality – the sort that can roll with the punches and take everything in their stride. When fate deals a hard knock they are philosophical, and rather than deny or suppress the truth, they seek to learn from the experience; somehow they manage to find the silver lining in every situation. They're the sort of people who are a joy to be around, striving for balance in all things. Because of their positive outlook, they rarely suffer mental health problems. They're extremely considerate of others but also take good care of themselves.
- **'Rajasic' people** have strong natural energy but very often 'burn out' because they do not know their limits and

are always excessively active and busy. Their minds are always racing, and switching off is nigh-on impossible. They are fiercely competitive and won't let anything or anyone stand in the way of their goals – which means they're also prone to being domineering. This hunger to progress also makes them impatient and inconsistent in their behaviour; prone to lashing out at others whom they blame for their problems, they very rarely accept blame themselves. While rajasic types often achieve their goals, they are lacking in spiritual awareness and purpose – so once the goals are achieved, they end up feeling empty, and this brings them great sorrow.

This lack of spiritual awareness can also bring them big shocks in life. Rather than having a belief in fate and accepting that good comes with bad, they seek for everything to go their way; when it doesn't, they can become angry, aggressive and increasingly disillusioned and depressed.

- 'Tamasic' types are repressed – a psychologist would say they have very deep-rooted issues that have never been dealt with in any way – they simply accept their 'lot' in life without considering that things could be better. Their energy is stagnant: they have no get up and go, and plod through life with little sense of purpose or enjoyment. They would not dream of seeking treatment or of talking to others about their feelings, and generally take poor care of themselves. Hygiene may be lacking.

While the types described above seem disparate, the truth is that we can all fluctuate between the states at different times in our lives. Given the frenetic energy of modern life, most of us will find ourselves within the rajasic bracket more often than not. The goal is, of course, to imbue our lives, minds, selves with sattva – and be able to live in a beautifully balanced way that brings peace, harmony and contentment.

The easiest way to begin one's journey toward sattva is by adopting a diet of mainly sattvic foods, with some energizing rajasic food, and even less stabilizing, nourishing tamasic food. Nothing is off-limits: it is, again, all about the right balance!

When formulating the gunas and guidelines, ancient Ayurvedic practitioners made a point of saying that for those who had to 'live in the world' – i.e. do jobs that required an energized state (as opposed to being a solely spiritual being) – it's necessary to eat rajasic food, but one must always be careful to balance this excitement out with sattvic foods.

Sattvic Foods

- Light and easy to digest – do not tax or burden the body
- Promote a feeling of contentment
- Bring mental clarity
- Full of 'prana' – life's energy. Food that is as fresh as possible, organic, seasonal, unprocessed
- Whole foods brimming with natural enzymes

Examples

Fruit: coconut, fig, mango, peach, pear, pomegranate
Veg: lettuce, parsley, sprouts, yellow squash, sweet potato
Grains: blue corn, basmati rice, tapioca
Beans: butter/lima, kidney, yellow split lentils, mung
Dairy: fresh whole organic milk, fresh homemade yogurt
Meat: none

Rajasic Foods

- Naturally stimulating
- Hot, spicy, salty and very sweet foods are all rajasic
- Foods that tempt are often rajasic
- Tea, coffee, chocolate, eggs and salt

Examples

Fruit: apples (particularly sour apples), bananas, guava
Veg: aubergines/eggplants, broccoli, cauliflower, capsicum peppers, potatoes, spinach, winter squashes, tamarinds, tomatoes
Grains: buckwheat, corn, millet, spelt
Beans: adzuki, red lentils, tur dal (also known as pigeon pea or gunga pea)
Dairy: sour cream
Meat: chicken, fish, prawns/shrimp

Tamasic Foods

- In moderation, grounding and stabilizing
- Too much causes lethargy – the sort of food that you need to sleep off!
- Feels heavy and makes us feel leaden
- Food that is past its best or stale is also tamasic
- Fermented 'vinegary' foods, and 'fungi' food – mushrooms and blue cheese, are all tamasic
- Alcohol and tobacco are tamasic

Examples

Fruit: apricots, avocados, plums
Veg: garlic, mushrooms, onions, pumpkins
Grains: brown rice, wheat
Beans: black beans, black lentils, pinto
Dairy: cheese
Meat: beef, lamb, pork

When you look at these lists, you should start to make links between the food you eat, your mood and your outlook. To feel truly, wonderfully balanced, it's important to eat food that best supports your dosha – and your sense of self.

eight

INNER BALANCE EQUALS OUTER GLOW

When we balance our diet, our guts and our digestion, wellbeing will certainly follow suit. But Ayurveda is about more than just the body. It is motivated by the mind, the soul, the spirit – and while the food that we eat has enormous impact on all of these, in order to feel truly balanced, we must work to unite both the internal and external. While I draw on Ayurveda in all I do, I also call upon other ideologies – ways of living that support Ayurveda and have offered me a great deal of support when I've needed it. Drawing upon nature's cures is at Ayurveda's core, but the use of flower essences isn't commonplace. It is, however, something that can really help us in our everyday lives, so I've also chosen to share it with you. A lot of us are familiar with the 'rescue remedy' type flower essence. One example is the catch-all remedy that alleviates panic and stress when dropped onto the tongue; I've been using it for many years and it's helped with everything from exams to childbirth! Flower essences go much further than these simple 'rescue' concoctions. They work by restoring the body's subtle energy flow – you may be familiar with the term 'chakra', which denotes the seven energy centres of the body, from the crown chakra (head) to the root chakra (base of the spine).

This chapter also looks at how knowledge of Ayurveda can affect our skin for the better. Over the years, I have found that simply being aware of how my dosha affects my skin keeps it calm, happy, balanced and beautiful. As Pitta, heat does not do me any favours, so I never take very hot baths or showers; I rinse my face with cool water, I don't use heat-up masks or abrasive exfoliants, or anything that is too 'active'. My skin just won't tolerate it.

I am fascinated by skin, by its responses and 'moods'. Shortly after the birth of my first child I decided to train as a holistic facialist. Having spent over a decade researching, trialling, testing and writing about skincare, health and wellbeing products (alongside experiencing myriad treatments, rituals and regimes), my interest in our bodies, and primarily our skin, had been irrevocably ignited. I reached a point where I no longer wanted to simply write about wellbeing; I wanted to be a purveyor of it too. My holistic facials begin on the inside, with an in-depth consultation that takes into account every part of the individual – from diet through to sleeping patterns, skin sensitivity to recent emotional trauma. Your skin is rather like a signpost: it displays the internal, external, emotional, psychological and physical passage of your life. There is almost always a reason behind the skin's signals, and learning to read them is both important and empowering – and crucial for helping us maintain our body's perfect balance.

For Ayurvedic skin advice, I've consulted Sunita Passi, the highly respected founder of Ayurvedic skincare brand Tri-Dosha, which is made with organic ingredients, including therapeutic Ayurvedic herbs. Here Sunita and I share five essential tips for incorporating Ayurveda into your beauty regime.

Five Steps to Balanced and Beautiful Skin

1. Observe Your Dosha

The fundamental goal of Ayurvedic practice is to maintain your own innate doshic balance – and that is the fundamental goal of this book, too! Knowing your dosha can also inform our beauty choices. It's particularly helpful when it comes to cleansing and moisturizing as every dosha has a very specific type of skin, and responds well to particular products.

As I feel it's important to use things that are as close to nature as possible, I often recommend the following:

- **For Vata**: soak a cosmetic sponge in raw milk, or live yogurt, and use it to cleanse the skin and pores. Rinse well. Milk and yogurt contain lactic acid, the wonderfully gentle exfoliant, hydrator and soother, so this works a treat as a cleanser.
- **For Pitta**: Coconut oil is a fantastic cleanser – simply warm it between your hands to melt, then massage over the face. It removes all make-up brilliantly. Remove with a warm, damp cloth.

- **For Kapha**: When skin is especially oily or congested, use a mix of apple cider vinegar, lemon or lime juice to remove oils and debris from the skin, and also to balance the skin's acid mantle, helping to keep the complexion healthy and clear.

2. Ayurvedic Therapy Needn't be Expensive

Simple, age-old Indian wisdom can help you acquire naturally glowing skin using herbal remedies made from ingredients you can find in your own home. A rummage around your kitchen is all you need for a lustrous complexion.

- **For Vata**: Combine cooked split orange lentils with ghee and milk until thickened into a paste. Apply as a deeply nourishing face mask and leave for five minutes. Remove with warm water.

- **For Pitta**: Mix turmeric powder and ground sandalwood in two teaspoons of milk to form a paste. Very high in antioxidants and soothing antihistamines, this combination is ideal for Pitta complexions, which can flare up easily. Apply to skin in a light coat and leave on for five minutes. Rinse away with warm water.

- **For Kapha**: In a blender or food processor, mix two tablespoons of plain yogurt with a kiwi fruit and one tablespoon each of almond oil, orange water and honey. The combination of exfoliating enzymes from the kiwi, hydrating lactic acid from the yogurt and nourishing and soothing orange water and honey make this a wonderfully balancing treat. Smooth over the face. After five minutes, remove with a warm wet cloth.

3. Turbo-charge Your Cosmetics with Massage

The power of touch, stretch (particularly within yoga) and massage are all important principles in Ayurveda. We so often look to others to help us when in fact we are already in possession of the only tools we need: our hands. If you do not already carry out facial massage, it's time to start.

I've met with two octogenarian Ayurvedic and yoga gurus in my time, both of whom had skin that was as supple and toned as that of a 40 year old. Their secret, they told me, was daily deep-tissue facial massage, which stimulates the nerve endings, in turn stimulating and toning up the facial muscles. It also boosts blood circulation, and any tissue that has blood coursing through it will be better oxygenated, more vital, radiant and healthy. Here is how to carry out a simple routine, which lasts five minutes, and should be repeated every morning:

- Place both thumbs under your chin, and the pads of your index and ring fingers in the space between your lower lip and your chin.
- You want to draw your hands out in long, smooth sweeping motions, with fingers pressed firmly but gently into the skin, and always stroking outward and upward,

toward the ears and temples. Let your fingers move firmly along the jawbone, as this is the area that is often most in need of firming.

- When your fingers reach the outside of the face, by the ears, circle the lobes with your thumb and index fingers, which is wonderfully soothing.
- Continue to sweep fingers all the way up the face, one inch at a time, and when you reach the eyes, stay below the orbital bone, massaging skin outward and upward toward the temples. When you reach the temples, press your index fingers lightly into the soft tissue there. Press and release slightly without breaking contact with the skin, for 10 seconds.
- Continue the same motion, upward and outward, over and above the brows, then from the centre of the brows, upward and outward over the forehead.
- Finish with fingers at the temples again – press and release as before, for another 10 seconds.
- Repeat the process five times.

4. Make Friends with Oil

If you want your body to run smoothly, you need to take oil both internally and externally. I take a blend of omega 3, 6 and 9 oils (see Resources, page 220), either straight off the spoon or drizzled over salads, into soups – you name it. If my eczema threatens to flare up, I take three tablespoons a day, every day for six weeks, and it usually settles down again. Topical application of oil is also essential. I've never been a body cream fan, preferring essential fatty-acid-rich oils. It's also easier to find 100 per cent organic oils as they don't need to be processed or fiddled with, thinned, thickened or coloured. They are what they are.

Neem oil is a wonderful antibacterial oil, ideal for dry, scaly skin – and great as a scalp treatment if you're prone to psoriasis or dandruff. It's always used in dilution (at no higher than 5 per cent concentration) as it's very potent and pungent. It can be bought in ready-to-use concentrations from most health shops or online.

In general, for everyday moisturising, Ayurveda recommends:

- **For Pitta**: Coconut oil, as it is inherently calming and cooling.
- **For Vata**: Sesame oil, which nourishes, warms and grounds (in Ayurveda it's also recommended as a perfect massage medium for irritable babies – rub into the soles of their feet before bedtime, where it will warm through them and help loosen the tension in the body. You can try it on yourself too).
- **For Kapha**: Sunflower oil is recommended, as it heats up the body, dispelling dampness and energizing the system.

All of the above options are cheap and effective, but I like to alternate with specially blended dosha-specific body oils – you can find these via internationally available brands Aveda and Tri-Dosha, Banyan Botanicals in the US and Ayurda in Australia and New Zealand.

5. Heal Problem Skin with Ayurveda

Ayurveda might be gentle but it's got serious skincare clout. Use the wisdom of Ayurveda to target specific skin problems such as blemishes and breakouts. Here are three age-old solutions to clear stubborn spots.

- **Make a herbal blemish paste**: Use water to make a paste using one teaspoon each of sandalwood powder and turmeric. Apply to your skin and leave for 15–20 minutes. Rinse off with lukewarm water. Do this daily until acne starts to subside.
- **Apply aloe vera**: Break open a leaf, take out the fresh gel, apply to your face and massage in. Once dry, wash off with lukewarm water. This formula does not cure acne but has amazing anti-inflammatory properties, helping to reduce the swelling and redness of pimples and acne. You will see results within a week.
- **Drink aloe vera**: Drinking aloe vera juice can enhance the vitality of the skin and is also useful in helping to alkalize and settle the stomach – Ayurveda believes that many skin problems originate in an unhealthy gut.

Ayurveda and Living Well

Aside from being a leading homeopath, Margo Marrone, the founder of the pioneering Organic Pharmacy, is also a font of wellness knowledge – the organic oracle, a seasoned homeopath and someone who also understands how tough it can be to juggle the demands of a very busy life (which she leads, with two kids and a booming international business) while maintaining a balanced body and clear mind. She's a big fan of the springtime detox and here imparts her tips for living well. They chime very neatly with many of Ayurveda's key principles, but they also focus on leading as organic a lifestyle as possible – something which isn't spelled out in Ayurveda, because it predates our use of chemicals and pesticides so food was always organic! For this reason, I think it crucial to couple an Ayurvedic lifestyle with both seasonal and organic living. The former just won't be 'balanced' unless it's supported by the latter. I've put many of Margo's suggestions into practice over the years (for myself and my children) and always feel so much better for having done so.

Top 10 Rules for Living Well

Margo Marrone

1 Eat consciously and think about everything you put inside your body – especially its health and nutrition value. Choose organic wherever you can to avoid toxic pesticides, hormones and antibiotics (particularly in soya, meat and dairy). Visit your local farmers' market for seasonal, fresh organic produce.

2 Your skin is an extension of your gut and what you put on it is just as important as what you eat. Your skin absorbs molecules small enough to penetrate the dermis. Lots of

cosmetics that we apply to the skin contain chemicals that are not healthy and can not only cause allergies but can even lead to a toxic overload of our systems – which in turn can cause chronic illnesses and disease, such as cancer. Always look for natural, organic plant-based products – the fewer preservatives, synthetics, fillers and harsh chemicals (particularly pthalates, sulphates and parabens) the better.

3   Feed your cells an abundance of antioxidants from vegetables and fruit, alongside a great antioxidant supplement. You need these to protect your cells and keep you young. Start when you are a teenager (ideally 15), and be religious about it. Most of the antioxidants that you take go to the vital organs in the body – the skin gets very little, so it also pays to apply antioxidant-rich cosmetics to your skin where they can act locally and ward off free radicals that are in UV and pollution.

4   Nourish your cells from within with essential fatty acids – essential to our health! If you have dry skin a tablespoon of omega oil every day is vital to restore elasticity. I recommend a blend of omega 3, 6, 7 and 9 – but at the very least, do increase both 3 and 6 intake.

5   The single most healing thing you can do is to detox your body. Not only does it lower stress, reduce bloating, sort out the digestion and improve sleep and performance, but it also gives the sort of energy you thought you would never have again. Do it gradually and gently four times a year and for at least 10 days – but make sure you eat healthily the entire time too.

6   If there is one thing to remove from your diet, it's sugar! Not only is it fattening, but it's also ageing (it causes cellular inflammation, which makes collagen and elastin break down faster). Sugar from fruit is fine in moderation (and best eaten on an empty stomach), but refined sugar should only be eaten rarely (or even better, never!).

7   Drink up – we are lucky to have access to 'clean' tap water but with industrialization come pesticides and other contaminants in our water system, including heavy metals and hormones. Either buy pure bottled water (in glass, as chemicals from the plastic bottles also pass into the water) or, better still, have a filter installed to remove these from your water before you drink or cook with it.

8   Scrub up well with a daily skin brush or body scrub to boost circulation and help the body eliminate toxins and better deliver nutrients to cells. Body brushing also stimulates the lymphatic system which helps keep you and your immune system clean and your skin baby soft.

9   Magnesium is a mineral that many people are lacking. Re-mineralize your body with an Epsom salt bath (follow the instructions on the packet) at least twice a week and take a magnesium complex supplement – particularly if you are stressed, exercise regularly and have problems relaxing or sleeping. Magnesium is the mineral world's tranquillizer (but without side effects!).

10 Inflammation is the body's way of keeping our health in check, but keep your skin and immune system's responses under control with daily doses of quercetin, vitamin C,

113

turmeric and bromelain (the enzyme from pineapples) – and of course avoid excessive sugar.

Ayurveda and Yoga

Yoga and Ayurveda are inseparable 'sister sciences', and both part of the wider Vedic science from which Ayurveda originates. I have enlisted the advice of a close friend and wonderfully spiritual yoga teacher, Selda Enver Goodwin. A big believer in Ayurveda (she is very Vata!), here she shares simple-to-master problem-solving poses. Please do try them – they will make an enormous difference to your wellbeing and your sense of inner balance.

Four Essential Yoga Poses to Find Body Balance

Selda Enver Goodwin

1. To Improve Sleep
Little frustrates me as much as a bout of insomnia. The body tosses, the mind ticks and muscles twitch. It's primarily caused by an increase in Vata in the mind or nervous system. It can also be related to constipation, stress and being over-tired. Oddly enough, getting out of bed can actually help.

Try Shoulder-stand pose at the end of the day, before bed or in the wee hours. It stimulates the thyroid, increases blood supply and soothes the nervous system, making it perfect for a calming night's rest. Avoid doing this during menstruation and late stages of pregnancy.

Lie on your back, and bend and squeeze your knees into your chest. With hands by your side, palms down, breathe out and raise your hips off the floor. Press your hands on your hips by bending your arms at the elbows. Breathe in. Raise the trunk up perpendicularly, supported by your hands until your chest touches your chin. If you suffer from high blood pressure, stay here and continue to breathe. Use your legs to balance you – bent or straight, whichever feels most comfortable. Only the back of the head and neck, the shoulders and the backs of the arms up to the elbows should rest on the floor. Place your hands to the middle of your spine, with your palms against your back. Breathe. Stretch your legs up to the sky, toes together, pointing up. Stay here for 5–10 minutes, with deep, even breaths. Gradually slide down, using your hands as support, then release and relax.

If you are a beginner, start by bending the right knee and placing the right foot on the left knee. Rotate or twist your hips forward to bring the knee to the forehead. The left leg should be horizontal to the floor. Repeat on the other side.

While I am in Shoulder-stand I imagine a tube of light running along my spine. I visualize my in- and out-breaths flowing up and down the tube. This creates focus and an intention for the breath to become louder than your thoughts.

115

2. To Boost Immunity

Health is an old English word for whole. Our immune system does a remarkable job in defending us against sickness, but on occasion even this miraculous structure weakens. Boosting immunity begins by understanding the immune system as a whole. Through yoga, we can balance and harmonize the entire body. Like many people, my body has a mini breakdown during the winter. I now take extra care to ensure that my body is insulated from within and my vitamin D levels are elevated. Then I formulate a physical and spiritual practice to protect my body at this time. Most yoga poses will help to increase your immunity, but one of my favourite poses for firing up the system is the Bridge. This posture is not only great for opening the area around the heart, it also presses directly on two main acupressure points. You'll get a feeling of vitality in the lower back and support on the shoulder blades, two inches away from the spine. These are the points said to help govern immunity, especially to colds and flu.

Lie on your back. Bend both knees and place your feet under your knees, hip-distance apart and parallel. Plant your hands by your hips and, curling your tailbone up to engage the navel, lift your hips high. Work your shoulder blades underneath you so they're flat on the floor, and if possible, reach for, or toward, the outside of your ankles. Do not bind the hands under your body as this can lift you onto your arm muscles, and off your shoulder blades. We want to focus on the pressure points there, and into the lower back. Lift your chin and arch your neck just enough so you could slip a hand between the back neck curve and the floor. If this is hard for you, place a high block or a rolled towel or two under your hips.

Stay here, breathing into the shoulder blades for one minute or more, then come down and gently hug your knees into your chest.

For a spiritual focus, I concentrate on lifting my heart up toward the sky and expanding my chest to opposite sides of the room. This actively increases the backbend, which is said to help us let go of our past and move us confidently into the future.

3. To Aid Digestion

When my digestion is out of sync, it's not just a 'gut feeling', it's my gut actually feeling bad. I'm prone to sudden skin breakouts and an overall body heaviness. I need to untangle the physical and emotional knots of life, often held in the belly region. I find Twists enhance the energy flow and nourish the organs back to full health. However, there are contraindications associated with going into deeper Twists, so it's best to start off with a very gentle body fold. In time, if you are not pregnant and not suffering from any back problems, hernia or hyperthyroidism, you can practise them under the guidance of a competent teacher.

For a simple, effective starter, lie on your stomach with interlaced fingers under your head. Bend the left leg sideways and bring your knee toward the ribs. Keep the right leg straight. Swivel your arms to the left, resting the left elbow near the left knee. Place the head on the elbow crease of the right arm or where it is comfortable. Rest here and take five full deep breaths, before changing sides.

While in this pose (which resembles a flapping fish), focus on the abdominal region. With as much detail as possible, I try to visualize the sensation running through and around my stomach. If it's feeling rather like sluggish dark molasses, I simply imagine golden liquid moving fluidly and freely from one organ to another. Visualization often helps to focus your attention and keeps your mind from racing back and forth. It does take time, so be patient and try not to punish yourself if everyday thoughts do take over. Acknowledge them, come back to the breaths and start over. It's called practice, after all.

4. To Combat Stress

Stress is difficult to define. What appears to be stressful for one individual is simply not so for another. This makes it more complicated to measure how much stress a person feels when exposed to certain situations. In yoga, we try to tap into our 'inner guru', or inner teacher. Listening to our bodies can often indicate the area that is causing stress. I have found that being open to experiencing the stress allows space for growth. I question, become aware of what it is that is happening and try to understand what my body is really feeling. I ask myself if it's fact or simply my interpretation. Is it my body or my mind that is doing the talking? Coming from a place of honesty or authenticity allows for shifts and transformation to take place. A method I use for achieving complete relaxation is Yoga Nidra or 'yoga sleep'. It can be practised any time of the day.

Lie down on your back on the floor, with a slight distance between the legs and both hands away from the thighs. The fingers of the hands should be open, palms facing the sky. Eventually the goal is to make the body become entirely still – peaceful, attentive; you get rest without becoming sluggish. Lie absolutely straight. Concentrate on the breath moving in and out of the body. Watch the body as the navel rises toward the sky during the inhalation and falls toward the earth on the exhalation. Experience the sensations of how the body is feeling as more breath comes into the lungs. Imagine them expanding, filling with air, light and vitality.

Then focus on one part of the body; perhaps start with the feet. Imagine your mind's eye looking at the toes, the big toes, the balls of the feet and the heels. Now make them absolutely loose. Move from the big toes to the ankles, the thighs, toward the abdomen, chest and eventually the head and the eyes. Tell each body part in turn to soften and just let go. In my experience, the first five to eight minutes can be the most challenging. The mind can be agitated and unsettled. Once this phase passes, the mind tends to calm and the thoughts slow down.

How Flower Essences Can Help us Find Balance

Flower essences are prepared by infusing the blossoms of plants in water, which is then diluted in a specific way and preserved. These preparations embody the distinct imprint or energetic pattern of each flower species, yet they differ from essential oils because they have no scent. The essences work through the body's acupuncture meridians, creating positive effects on the way we feel, and are a vibrational tool that helps people reach their full potential.

Once you get used to using flower essences, you'll see how effectively they work to harmonize your system and offer real strength and solace at times when you're really struggling. A flower essence, however, is only as good as its producer, and the homogenized bottled ones you get in most big supermarket-style pharmacies might have been on the shelf for years, gathering dust and depreciating the entire time. Try to find a reputable organic essence provider – the internet is a great source of organically certified producers who work with tiny batches, and can ensure quality. If in doubt, testimonial pages can really help you make up your mind.

Here's a list of some of Annee de Mamiel's favourite flower essences to provide you with a powerful alternative therapy kit.

Top Six Flower Essences for Balance

Annee de Mamiel

- **Aloe vera** flower essence is needed by those burning the candle at both ends. These individuals may tend to overuse their innate abundance of fiery forces, resulting in burnout. Typical users of aloe vera are workaholic types whose drive is so intense that they neglect their emotional and physical needs, often sacrificing rest, food and social contact in order to accomplish their goals.

- **Alpine aster** is great whenever you find it difficult to rest and relax, feeling cut off from your core, constantly on the go, for busy times full of stimulus/worry/excitement – when you have little time to connect within. It helps create time for contemplation and review; for retreat and recuperation.
- **Fig** releases fears, improves memory and helps you to organize your thoughts.
- **Le jardin des alpes** encourages rest, renewal and relaxation. It helps you let go of external demands for a period in order to return to gentleness and compassion within. It helps you to be present and find renewal in the everyday rather than waiting for some imaginary time in the future when you hope you will be able to stop and be still.
- **Nasturtium** is powerful and begets glowing vitality, flaming, radiant energy and warmth, new possibilities, inspiration and courage.
- **Rosemary** imparts a warm physical presence, clarity of perception, memory and a richer, higher perspective.

nine

HOW TO BALANCE THE GOOD WITH THE 'BAD'

When I started writing this chapter, I gave it the title, 'Why Guilt (Not Chocolate) Makes Us Fat'. I really do believe that the stress and worry and guilt we lay upon ourselves are the biggest contributing factor to weight gain in the modern world. I also realize that if you do little other than eat fries, chocolate and cake, then it's unlikely you'll have a balanced, slim body! As you'll know if you've read this far, I also believe that we're often eating for a myriad of reasons that have absolutely nothing to do with actual hunger. Aside from commonplace (and already discussed) emotional eating, or comfort eating, there's another approach to tackling this food stress that is unique to Ayurveda.

When I first began my Ayurvedic journey, I learned that some of the foods that weren't doing me any favours were my *trigger* foods – there's a fair bit of food we eat that imbalances our dosha, and we eat it for emotional rather than appetite-related reasons. One of the Ayurvedic gurus I met with suggested this was a subconscious form of self-harm . . . now I wouldn't go that far, but I think we've all felt that 'I've had a crap day so I'm going to eat really crap food' feeling.

The Body Balance Plan, however, is about exorcising that feeling once and for all. Guilt has no place within our diet, because the moment we feel guilty or stressed about food, we produce cortisol, a hormone which actually prevents us from losing weight.

One of the UK's leading nutritionists, Eve Kalinik, says, 'cortisol is a hormone used by the body to stimulate fat and carbohydrate metabolism for fast energy. It also stimulates insulin release and the maintenance of blood sugar, which increases appetite, so ordinarily you would feel the need to consume more. The problem with disrupting the usual rhythm of cortisol secretion is that it promotes weight gain and fat deposition – particularly around the middle area. Cortisol is produced by the adrenal glands, which are part of the endocrine system that includes the thyroid, which is responsible for managing metabolic rate. An increase in circulating cortisol has a direct inhibitory affect on thyroid activity, which means that metabolic rate is slowed and therefore weight loss is more difficult. You may even see a weight gain despite consuming the same amount of calories. That's why when I work with clients who are trying to lose weight without success I often address their adrenal function before looking at anything else.'

Given that this is a health book, I am about to say something controversial.

Sometimes we'll want to dig into a tub of chocolate ice cream. Sometimes we'll want to polish off a packet of Maltesers while watching a bad movie. Sometimes we'll want to order a grande caramel latte (even when we know how many calories are in it). I think this is okay – I really do. Because sometimes we have to be able to just eat or drink precisely what it is that we fancy, even when it's not going to nourish us nutritionally. It's nourishing us in other ways – if you enjoy it, really want it, and have it at the right time. Food can be about guilt-free indulgence, enjoyment, deliciousness – every now and again.

I strongly believe it's far more damaging, and potentially dangerous in the long term, to swear off sweet 'bad' foods forever. By doing that, you're making them more powerful than they are, and you subsequently need to expend a lot of energy trying to avoid them and deny them to yourself, every day for the rest of your life. My slimmest, happiest, healthiest friends have this attitude to food. Yes, I eat very healthily, in a balanced, nourishing, seasonal way 85 to 90 per cent of the time, but I will dig into that delicious sticky toffee pudding, or enjoy the bowl of organic ice cream that sings with scrumptiousness in the summer. Because nothing is off-limits, I don't ever need to 'worry' about food.

When it goes beyond the 'once in a while', it becomes something else – a crutch, a comfort, a way of punishing or rewarding ourselves – and food has no place in this cycle. When we eat mindlessly, when we eat because we're stressed and the adrenalin rush we're on tells us we need sugar and fat (we don't), or when we don't really want it, eat far more of it than we actually enjoy, go back for seconds when we're already full, or just eat something because it's there, at the wrong time, when we know we actually fancy something completely different – that's when it's just a waste of food, a waste of our own internal energy, and also saps our sense of wellbeing. We're also likely to feel most guilty about food when we eat in this way, with that empty feeling that lingers on, long after we've filled ourselves with the wrong food.

When to Check the Label

No, this is not about calorie counting. But there's a reason why everyone should be food-label savvy, and that's to avoid the mass of unnecessary additives which are pumped into food that ought, in fact, to be very, very simple. A key part of Ayurveda – and any sensible diet – is to eat food 'that's as close to nature as possible'. While we're not all going to subsist on fruit and veg that's just been plucked from the plant, there's merit in eating things that have undergone as few processes as possible.

Bread

Bread is my number one bugbear. I know we don't all have time to bake (my husband and I often go weeks without finding the time), but we can look for bread that is baked fresh and sold fresh (not part-baked, frozen, stored, transported and shelved – bread that is bleached, refined, sugared, salted and overly yeasty). And that's just the beginning. To find out more about the 'invisible' things added to bread that legally do not even have to appear on the label, you might want to visit www.sustainweb.org/realbread, run by a collective of food enthusiasts and part of the charity Sustain – the alliance for better food and farming – which kickstarted the Real Bread Campaign. It makes for pretty sobering reading!

Like Sustain, I think we should all follow the lead of the French, who actually have a bread law, which clearly states which ingredients are permissible (no artificial additives, only wheat bread flour, drinkable water, cooking salt; the only permissible added extras are 2 per cent bean meal, 0.5 per cent soya bean meal and 0.3 per cent malted wheat flour). It also states that at no point during the bread's making can it be frozen, and that if it's called 'fresh' or 'homebaked' (*pain maison*) it must actually have been kneaded, shaped and baked in the place where it is also finally sold to the customer.

So, when it comes to shop-bought bread, always, always use your loaf! And, considering that Brits ate 1.69 billion sandwiches last year (according to the British Sandwich Association) and Americans eat 300 million sandwiches every day, or 109.5 billion a year, such a staple part of the convenience diet really does need a second look (and label check), every time.

The irony is that unprocessed food always tastes far better than processed food – we're just used to eating things that are convenient and consequently messed around with. In my home we eat organic butter because we're put off by all the freaky things that go into making margarine so spreadable. Even the organic margarines are processed in the sense that ingredients like water and palm fat are added to sunflower oil to make it thicker. If margarine tasted lovely that would be one thing, but it's got nothing on butter spread on a piece of steaming fresh hot bread. Lately, I've also discovered the yumminess that is fresh toasted bread spread with raw coconut oil (solid at room temperature, it's like an opaque white butter). It gives the toast a lovely subtle coconutty taste, which is wonderful with honey on top, or, even better, my Wholesome Speedy Nutty Butter (see the recipe on pages 176–7).

Make Good Choices – Listen to Your Body

This brings me to another core part of the Body Balance Plan: I believe that every food choice needs to be, on some level, a wise choice. You want to eat something deliciously sweet and chocolaty, but that hydrogenate-filled week-old-but-still-freakishly-soft cupcake is a poor runner-up to that steaming hot fresh-baked additive- and preservative-free chocolate muffin made by a friend (or a good local bakery). Our bodies and minds can only thrive if fed with good stuff. I'm not anti-sugar, anti-fat, anti-anything, aside from anti-empty-rubbish-fake-food which never satiates and never nourishes.

I do eat sugar – despite the many research-backed studies that link a diet high in sugar to all sorts of problems, including an increased risk of depression. But I also believe that entirely depriving ourselves of something is unhealthy too, and certainly risks fostering an imbalanced attitude toward food. I go ahead and continue to enjoy chocolate and cake, but I try to 'balance' these things with very nutritious, fresh, seasonal, antioxidant-, mineral- and vitamin-rich food.

I do, however, have standards – even with the sweet stuff. Those E-number-filled cakes and sweets/candies fool us into thinking we want them, but once we've eaten them, we feel empty – and often jittery and hungrier soon after as a result of the high sugar content of the 'food'. By all means have your cake and eat it (and your ice cream and your chocolate too), but always, always, be aware of what it is you're putting into your body.

It can take a bit of time to get used to decoding what your body needs – most commonly, the moment we need energy we crave sugar or caffeine, which, admittedly, isn't going to do us any long-term good. But we all know that 4pm urge well (at work, we call it 'Biscuit-Tin Time'); when lunch is fully digested and the body begins to run out of energy reserves, we hanker after a pick-me-up and it's often chocolate-bar shaped. I'll be the first to admit to being very familiar with that craving. I adore chocolate – the way it melts on the tongue, its inviting smell, those immediate endorphin highs you get when enjoying those first few squares – but I adopted several choc-craving rules almost a decade ago now, and though I continue to enjoy the stuff in all of its many guises, I always observe the following common-sense notions:

1. Never on an Empty Stomach

If I'm very hungry, eating any food that is high in refined sugar just makes me feel shaky and sick, so if I'm stuck at a station scrabbling for a snack before my train speeds off, I look for nuts, fruit, oatcakes, rye crackers or, if I'm lucky, those hummus and veggie pots instead.

2. Sweeten Your Tea

I discovered chyawanprash relatively recently – it's a commonly used blend of over 30 herbs, and is simultaneously sweet, sour and spicy. It's quite lovely – a thick, sticky jam texture, made primarily from the amla fruit, and very high in both antioxidants and dosha-reducing herbs. You can eat it off the spoon, but if, like me, you like your 'chai' – and are familiar with the cardamom, clove and cinnamon blend that often dominates it – then you'll certainly like this. As an experiment, for a week, every time I had a chocolate craving I stirred a half-teaspoon of this into a cup of hot rooibos tea and was delighted to find that, almost without fail, that interest in chocolate dissipated within seconds.

I believe this is because it's teaching the body to recognize 'sweet' in terms of what it needs (the Sweet taste, which also reduces Vata and Pitta), not the artificial sweetness of sugar which provides energy but no vitamins, minerals or antioxidants. This is great to keep in the desk drawer, and to sip on several times a day to keep the body balanced and sugar cravings in check.

3. Pick 'n' Mix

A few chocolate buttons (some dark, some milk, some white if you really want to indulge) mixed with a small handful of almonds, cashews, Brazils and some sugar-free organic cereal (I like spelt or oat bran flakes, or nick some of my daughter's organic multigrain cereal O's) is a better way to enjoy your chocolate than having a whole bar. It's far more satisfying, but still sweet. You're still eating the choc, so your brain gets what it wants, but the good stuff in between is what stops you eating more than you ought to. The mix of fibre and protein also keeps my blood sugar stable. Or, for a totally divine treat, dip your buttons into nut butter – utterly delicious, and with added protein.

4. Upgrade It

I regularly eat an early dinner (around 5pm) with the children, so I can become quite peckish again before bedtime (between 10 and 11pm). Instead of chomping on chocolate just before bedtime, which would simply send me into a downward refined-sugar spiral, I make my satiating and delicious Chia Choc Bars (see the recipe on pages 212–13) twice a week (they take under 10 minutes to mix and spoon into a baking tray, then 15 minutes to bake), and stash them in a Tupperware box, ready to accompany my nightly cup or two of tea (I drink naturally caffeine-free teas such as rooibos and fennel, mixed with a half-teaspoon of chyawanprash). I try not to eat anything for at least two hours before bedtime, though – I always sleep poorly and wake up bloated if I eat too much, too late.

5. Try Raw Chocolate

I once reviewed a raw food delivery diet company, and while I reached the conclusion that all raw food all the time wasn't doing my constitution any favours, I did fall utterly in love with their raw chocolate truffles. Raw chocolate (which is ordinarily mixed with cocoa butter and agave) really has its place because of the very high cocoa content, which makes it very high in antioxidants and still tastes pretty yummy. Now I like sweet milk chocolate, and I'm not going to pretend that raw chocolate can be mistaken for it, but once I'd had, and enjoyed, a raw chocolate truffle or two after dinner, I really didn't want 'normal' chocolate afterwards. So, for those of us who occasionally let our sugar cravings get the better of us – or just feel like we'd like to nip the chocolate habit in the bud – raw chocolate is a great alternative. Just be sure to look for good raw versions that substitute sugar for a healthier, low-GI, unprocessed, natural sweetener – jaggery is a great alternative (visit www.balanceplan.co.uk to find out more about the best Ayurveda-approved sweeteners and where to find them).

ten

WELCOME TO YOUR IMMERSION DIET AND THE BEGINNING OF A BALANCED BODY

Finding time to make any level of change is not easy. I know this first hand, as someone who feels lucky when I find myself with a (rare) couple of free hours in the evening, once essential life tasks are ticked off, children fed, enjoyed and put to bed and all work projects completed. So, I want to offer a realistic approach. Rather than asking that you take seven days (which is nigh-on impossible unless you take a complete holiday, and even then, if family or work commitments sneak in, you'll be forced to cut corners), I have built this immersion into three dedicated, restful days away from work and heavy responsibilities (perhaps over a long weekend) and I then adjust the plan to allow you to go back to work, but continue with your immersion at a realistic pace that will slot in and around your existing routine. Being able to take this time to yourself, and allow yourself true peace, rest and relaxation, will mean that your body is more powerfully supported and you'll achieve faster results.

This immersion is designed to work at any time of year alongside your general Ayurvedic diet (although doing it in spring does give you the mental edge, as we're wired to *want* a fresh start in spring), and is the perfect introduction for Ayurveda virgins, but also a great top-up – to boost immunity and energy or to cleanse the system after a period of not eating to plan.

Doing this immersion at home is also uniquely supportive of Ayurveda as you're disturbing as little of your life and routine as possible. Your home environment is naturally nurturing – it's familiar and safe, and embarking upon a lifestyle change at home (rather than in an expensive spa, or on a retreat across the other side of the world) gives you a real advantage. It means you don't have the classic 'Catch-22' of going away to make a 'fresh start' which falls by the wayside the moment you return home to 'real life'. While I first learned about Ayurveda on my retreat in the Maldives, it was some time before I was able to introduce Ayurveda properly into my home life. I was on a learning journey, and my interest was piqued, but until I sat down and started thinking about how to shop, cook and live it in the UK, it wasn't a real part of my life. This is why I always condone changes that start at home – you'll get a true insight into a new way of doing things that realistically fits around your family and existing environment.

The main focus of this plan is to shift stubborn ama. As we've discovered, ama is often the thing that prevents us from losing weight – this build-up of toxins and waste material is hard to cleanse. It requires a committed approach, and strategic use of certain herbs and spices, which all enable the body to steadily rid itself of this deeply stored stagnant matter. There are some 'best practice' options; if you can commit to doing them, please do – you'll feel so much better for it – or 'gentler' options, which will be less powerful, but still effective. Lest you start to panic, I can also assure you that nothing is aggressive.

Ayurveda is so beautifully in tune with life and the body that all change is seen as a result of organic rebalancing. We may be in possession of 'excesses' which need to be purged, but Ayurveda knows that an overly strict or spartan approach can cause further deficiencies. In order to balance, without taking too much away, or putting too much strain on the system, a specific blend of whole foods, herbs and spices is recommended. The good news is you never go hungry – it is a food-based cleanse that will nourish, uplift, soothe and calm, while also working to kickstart purification and cleansing of the digestive system (but without horrible side effects).

I know many people are advocates for all-raw or juice-only cleanses, and thankfully, Ayurveda does not endorse this approach. If you are attempting to cleanse your body it will need to be amply supported, and an all-raw diet is just too taxing to your digestion (and a bad idea in cold weather as it really increases Vata), while a juice-only diet is just not satiating enough (and hunger is the ultimate enemy of diet success, along with being the main cause of serious grumpiness on my part!). Being hungry also causes acute anxiety; we're conditioned to panic when food isn't available, and this is why crash dieting is doomed to fail. Feeling anxious, grumpy, even angry because you're hungry is not conducive to a mind/body cleanse. We want to discover balance and find peace – not spend a week dreaming about chocolate bars and big bowls of pasta.

As I found during my first immersion diet, many years ago now, I could still eat, and eat well, as long as food was appropriate and easily digested. I felt strong and vital, slept well, my skin brightened and, yes, I lost eight pounds in a week. My immersion was also amply supported by Ayurvedic treatments which focused on rebalancing my chakras, and if it's possible for you to enjoy an Ayurvedic treatment from a reputable practitioner during your immersion, I'd wholeheartedly recommend it. Again, the power of treating the outside along with the inside is always more powerful and promotes changes that are far more likely to 'stick'.

Alongside diet advice, there are some strong lifestyle and wellbeing suggestions. What I find most impressive (and intuitive) about Ayurveda is the understanding that, even when we're eating good food, we're not able to get from it what we need if our frame of mind or body isn't in the right place. If your stomach is in figurative knots, it's not going to do the best job of digesting what goes into it. Ayurveda understands the strain that stress, anxiety, fear, grief and so on can have upon the digestive system, and though we're certainly helping ourselves when we put in wholly nourishing, balanced food, we can't expect to be truly balanced until we put all of the emotional stresses and strains to rest too.

This plan, therefore, is designed to get us to a place where every part of our mind, body and gut is in optimal balance, and this is the place from where we can move forward, stronger and more vitally than would've been possible if we took a surface-only approach.

Before You Immerse Yourself . . .

1. I've found that it's always helpful to say things out loud – to yourself, and to those around you. If you have decided to embark upon this Ayurvedic immersion, you should tell your family and friends. It will give you permission to take the time and space you'll need to do it properly, and also cement your intention to make this change. Being supported by your partner or children can be a key part of this process – you may even find that a friend would like to try it alongside you. This is, however, a necessarily solitary exercise . . .

2. . . . so make time to be alone, peaceful and reflective. Including daily yoga into your routine is a great way to make this time. If yoga is entirely new to you, try to make the time for a class (if you want to stay at home, www. balanceplan.co.uk has wonderful quick, but effective yoga sessions to guide you in your practice). Journaling is another valid way of making 'me' time. Schedule 15

minutes into your day, the week before you begin, and write down your thoughts and feelings as they occur to you. It will help prepare your mind for the change it's about to encounter too.

3. Get as much rest as possible. Try to get your sleeping schedule on track, even if it means lights out at the same time every night. If you are always fidgety in bed and take an age to wind down, try an ancient Ayurvedic trick – deeply massage warm sesame oil into the soles of your feet before getting into bed. It will warm the body up and ease tension as you sleep.

4. Try to eat in line with your dosha for the days leading up to your immersion. It will start to bolster your body before you've even begun. It's also wise to cut down on the things you know aren't helping you – nicotine, caffeine, alcohol, refined foods and excess sugar.

The Three-Day Immersion

Choose three consecutive quiet days, when you have few commitments and you are not working. Surround yourself with things that encourage peace of mind and a sense of wellbeing: your favourite classical music, a cherished novel, some new watercolour paints to experiment with. This is your time – an Ayurvedic holiday of sorts. Try to start each day with optimism and joyful anticipation.

Day 1

1. After waking, drink a glass of hot water (you can add a slice of fresh ginger or a squeeze of lime; or add a cinnamon stick or a crushed cardamom pod, then strain) to hydrate and encourage cleansing.
2. Take time to massage your entire body with a dosha-specific oil (see page 109). Sesame oil can be used by all three doshas – its warming, nurturing properties are ideal for your body when it's going through a period of cleansing. For a step-by-step guide to Abhanga massage, be sure to visit www.balanceplan.co.uk.

3. Your first meal should be a nurturing porridge (see recipes on pages 173–6 for different porridge options, and choose the version that best supports your dosha). Ayurvedic puritans often make porridge with basmati rice (which is quite tasty) or dhal (which I find a bit strange for my palate), and I like to vary the grains I use to keep things interesting. Chia seeds, oats, quinoa and millet are all good, and I offer a variety in the recipe section.

4. Your lunch should be a balancing, cleansing dish that I call my Soul-Soothing Stew for its easy nourishing properties (see recipe on pages 194–5). Based on kitchari – the traditional healing Ayurvedic dish – it is designed to be eaten at times when the body is weak, needs repair, needs to detox and cannot be taxed. It is easily digested, tasty and filling. As I also believe that variety is important in terms of nourishing the body, I suggest some additional touches and flourishes to add interest to this dish if you are going to be on the immersion for several days.

5. Take an hour in the middle of the day to do some yoga.

6. If the weather is conducive, take a leisurely stroll outside – ideal in spring, summer or early autumn, when the weather is still mild. Take your time, breathe deeply and pay attention to your natural environment. If it's winter, bright clear days are also lovely for a walk, but I wouldn't recommend a stroll in very wet or bitterly windy weather – your body needs support, not a meteorological onslaught! If the weather is unwelcoming, it is still important to get some fresh air, so throw open the

windows of your home and let the fresh wind rip through for a few minutes; just ensure you're wrapped up. Do this every few hours to prevent the air in your home getting stagnant (especially important if you use central heating).

7. Dinner should be another small bowl of Soul-Soothing Stew (see pages 194–5).

8. Between 30 minutes and an hour before you plan to fall asleep, take two Triphala tablets with a glass of warm water. This will help the body cleanse itself further overnight, and also help combat potential constipation (although due to the natural whole foods you'll be eating it would very unusual to experience this on the immersion diet).

9. Dim the lights, turn off all electrical gadgets and choose a book for bedtime. Bathing at night isn't traditionally advised in Ayurveda, but I find nothing encourages sleep more effectively. Burn a favourite natural-wax, non-smoking candle as you run a bath. Add a big scoop of magnesium salts to the bath, let them dissolve, then sink into the water. I like to fill the bath just high enough to allow me to lie flat within it, water covering my ears and body, my nose and mouth just out of the water. The feeling of submerging the head is incomparably relaxing and great if you've felt slightly headachy today.

10. Massage your specific oil all over your body, pull on some comfortable cotton pyjamas and get into bed to read for 30 minutes, before turning the light out and going to sleep.

11. Keep a glass of room-temperature water by your bed as you may feel thirsty through the night as your body begins to purge excess salts and toxins.

Day 2

1. After waking, drink a glass of hot water (you can add a slice of fresh ginger or a squeeze of lime; or add a cinnamon stick or a crushed cardamom pod, then strain).

2. Half an hour after your water, enjoy a bowl of dosha-specific porridge, chosen from the recipe section.

3. Attend a morning yoga session – use a DVD, an online tutorial, or, if you have a nice local class that is within easy reach, find the time to attend today.

4. Lunch can be Soul-Soothing Stew, Love Broth or Red Lentil and Coconut Soup (see recipes on pages 194–5 and 199–202).

5. If it is summer and the weather is overly hot, enjoy a post-lunch siesta in a room with open windows. If it is winter, curl up under a warm blanket and rest for an hour, letting thoughts come into your mind freely, which you then acknowledge and release without focusing on them. Focus instead on your breathing and the feeling of release within your body.

6. Once you're rested, choose a favourite activity: some non-strenuous gardening, painting, reading, singing, listening to music. Concentrate on the task at hand, enjoying the

focus you give to it, and feel your breath slowing and steadying as you continue to relax.

7. Take time to prepare a nourishing supper – my Soul-Soothing Stew will continue to nourish you now. Feel free to add some extra, different vegetables that will also balance your dosha – courgette/zucchini and sweet potatoes are great for Vata and Pitta types, add cauliflower or beetroot for Kapha. You can also alter spicing to add interest – adding ground ginger for both Vata and Kapha, and coconut flakes or fresh coriander/cilantro leaves for Pitta.

8. Eat slowly, lovingly, without distraction.

9. Between 30 minutes and an hour before you plan to fall asleep, take two Triphala tablets with a glass of warm water. Again, this will help the body cleanse itself further overnight and also dispel excess gas and soothe the stomach.

10. Dim the lights, turn off all electrical gadgets and ready your book for bedtime. Take another mineralizing bath – add a big scoop of magnesium salts to hot water, let them dissolve, then sink into the bath.

11. Massage your specific oil all over your body, pull on some comfortable cotton pyjamas and get into bed to read for 30 minutes, before turning the light out and going to sleep.

12. Keep a glass of room-temperature water by your bed as you may feel thirsty through the night as your body purges excess salts and toxins.

Day 3

1. This is the last day of your immersion diet. Wake up with purpose, reflectively and meaningfully and consider all the things you are thankful for and that help put a smile on your face.

2. Drink a glass of hot water (you can add a slice of fresh ginger or a squeeze of lime; or add a cinnamon stick or a crushed cardamom pod, then strain).

3. Wait 30 minutes, then enjoy a bowl of nourishing dosha-specific porridge.

4. Curl up with your book and spend the morning reading, or if you prefer, journaling – writing down the thoughts you have as and when they occur to you. If any thoughts are negative or worrisome, think about what you may be able to do to resolve them throughout the course of the next week. Write down your resolutions and make a plan of action, then put it away in a drawer, ready to take out tomorrow, when your immersion will be over and you will feel even more energized.

5. Enjoy a steamed green vegetable salad for lunch. Choose from the recipes below according to your dosha type, and use organic vegetables. This is my Ayurvedic take on an alkalizing raw green juice, but it doesn't tax the body. Juicing is not recommended for Vata types, who need to eat warming, nourishing meals to keep their systems in check (juice fasts will make you gassy, irritable and uncomfortable). Pitta types too, because of their strong

digestive fire, needs to eat regular proper meals to sustain energy levels, not cut down to a few juices a day (this will do nothing to keep agni fired up either). Kapha types may be the only exception here, in that these types do well to fast occasionally, and will feel far more energized than the other doshas if they do.

- **For Vata**: Prepare (wash, peel, trim) one small courgette/zucchini, four spears of asparagus, one small leek and a small cucumber (English 'hothouse' cucumbers are much sweeter than ridge varieties). Chop into 2.5cm/1in-long pieces, and cook all but the cucumber through in a pan with some good olive oil and a pinch of Himalayan rock salt, plus parsley, poppy seeds, ground coriander and garlic, until all the vegetables begin to tenderize. Once tender, add the cucumber to warm through. Drizzle with sesame or olive oil, add a squeeze of lime and eat slowly, chewing every mouthful thoroughly.

- **For Pitta**: Prepare (wash, peel, trim) one small courgette/zucchini, four spears of asparagus, one small leek, a handful of broccoli florets and a small cucumber. Chop into 2.5cm/1in-long pieces, and cook all but the cucumber through in a pan with some good olive oil and a pinch of Himalayan rock salt, plus ground coriander, fresh ginger and fresh basil, until all the vegetables begin to tenderize. Once tender, add the cucumber to warm through. Drizzle with walnut or olive oil, add a squeeze of lime and eat slowly, chewing every mouthful thoroughly.

- **For Kapha**: Prepare (wash, peel, trim) one small artichoke heart, four spears of asparagus, one small leek, a handful of broccoli florets, and a handful of celery. Chop into 2.5cm/1in-long pieces, and cook through in a pan with some sunflower oil and a pinch of cayenne, plus ground ginger, fresh grated garlic and some poppy seeds, until all the vegetables begin to tenderize. Once tender, add a squeeze of lime and eat slowly, chewing every mouthful thoroughly.

6. Have a rest after lunch.
7. Attend an afternoon yoga class, or follow a DVD or an online tutorial.
8. Dinner can be Soul-Soothing Stew, Love Broth or Red Lentil and Coconut Soup (see recipes on pages 194–5 and 199–202).
9. Eat slowly, lovingly, without distraction.
10. Between 30 minutes and an hour before you plan to fall asleep, take two Triphala tablets with a glass of warm water. This will help the body cleanse itself further overnight and also dispel excess gas and soothe the stomach.
11. Dim the lights, turn off all electrical gadgets and ready your book for bedtime. Take another mineralizing bath – adding a big scoop of magnesium salts to hot water, let them dissolve, then sink into it.
12. Massage your specific oil all over your body, pull on some comfortable cotton pyjamas and get into bed to read for 30 minutes before turning lights out and going to sleep.

13. Keep a glass of room-temperature water by your bed as you may feel thirsty through the night as your body begins to purge excess salts and toxins.

For the rest of the week begin every day with hot water and some ginger, lime or cardamom. Continue to drink herbal teas and filtered water. Eat Ayurvedically as much as possible – the recipes at the back of this book will really help you.

Additional Notes

Drinks

You can drink any variety of herbal teas throughout the day – tulsi tea is a great tonic, elevating and balancing the mind and mood alongside supporting your cleansing system. Fennel, nettle, aniseed, sage and ginger tea are all good too. Check the Taste Table (on pages 153–64) to find out which teas best support your dosha. All the water you drink during the immersion should be warm (boil the kettle and get into the habit of using it to top up your filtered water with hot water throughout the course of the day).

Snacks

If at any point you feel hungry, try a cup of tea. If you are still hungry after the tea, prepare a light snack. Make it unprocessed whole food and dosha-specific – seasonal fruits, raw unsalted and unprocessed nuts, lightly steamed seasonal vegetables, or even a small extra helping of Soul-Soothing Stew if you are feeling particularly hungry. You could also make up a batch of Love Broth, a healing, nourishing soup that can be enjoyed in place of cups of tea if you get tea'd out! Do try not to eat for eating's sake, though – allowing the body to digest the food you eat for breakfast, lunch and dinner is important, and will be difficult if you snack all day. Likewise, don't feel you need to go hungry if you're getting genuine pangs. Be true to what you need and listen to your body – a key part of achieving body balance! If you're having trouble determining whether your hunger is 'real' or imagined, schedule a walk or one of the wellbeing suggestions below into the spaces between meals. If you're like me, you may well find that all you need for your hunger to dissipate is a bit of distraction.

Wellbeing

As this is your time, enjoy a few pampering Ayurvedic rituals such as the one opposite, all of which are aimed at aligning your chakras and achieving a sense of unity between body and mind.

What Comes After Your Immersion?

If you immerse yourself for three days, the main thing to try and hang onto is the sense of control and calm you'll gain from this focused 'you' time. It's so easy to get sucked back into the drama and pressure of 'real life' – and it goes without saying that real life will go on, with or without you – but there must be a way for you to assimilate all you've learned and experienced

Balancing the Chakras

Denise Leicester, founder of Ila Beauty

Music and massage are subtle ways to touch the most sensitive and vulnerable yet powerful parts of ourselves – the chakras. Bathing in a Himalayan salt bath with oils such as vetiver, spikenard, patchouli and a little ginger is very nurturing to the earth (*muladhara*) and water chakras (*swadhisthana*).

Chakras respond to healing music, especially certain mantras that have vibrational healing for the chakras.

Conscious massage is a beautiful way to nourish the heart chakra (*anahata*) as the skin and the hands are the organs that are connected to the heart. Oils such as jasmine, rose and sandalwood have a beautiful resonance with the heart. Acknowledging each part of the body with love and gratitude as you massage is wonderful.

Foot baths and reflexology are very healing to the solar plexus (*manipura*) chakra as the feet are organs connected to the solar plexus. The soul (*ajna*) and crown (*sahasara*) chakras are balanced through meditation and stillness.

into that daily routine. The main thing that will help you is the maintenance of a balancing, supporting, stress-relieving diet – this will be your food foundation, a strong helping hand to keep you healthy, even when life is more taxing than normal.

Acquaint yourself with the recipes in this book, and the Taste Table, and whenever possible try to choose a meal that will help support you and balance your dosha for at least a full week after your immersion. By eating Ayurvedically you'll continue to carry the torch lit during your immersion, and fan that digestive fire, which will continue to grow and flourish if you carry on taking in the correct food. By eating this way, as often as you can, you'll steadily find your body moving closer to its centre, and closer to its natural, balanced, healthy state.

Food is miraculous, but it is not the whole picture. In the days after your immersion, it's also important to continue to strive for peace of mind and clarity of purpose. You made the time to immerse yourself, you did something quite wonderful, something beautiful for your body – don't let it slip away. Every day after your immersion do a bit of yoga, meditate, practise mindfulness, carry out an Ayurvedic massage . . . or continue in an even more committed way by seeking out a local Ayurvedic centre or group, and begin to incorporate the seasonal wisdom of this incredible, ancient science into the circle of people you share your life with. Cooking for other Ayurveda lovers is really satisfying – a great learning curve and fantastic way to pick up new recipes yourself too. This book is just the beginning of what could become a naturally balanced way of life, for life.

The Taste Table

The very kind Ayurvedic Institute, run by world-renowned Ayurvedic physician Vasant Lad, BAMS, MASc, has here allowed me to reproduce their incomparably thorough Food Guidelines for Constitutional Types (which I've nicknamed the Taste Table). Nobody has ever done it better, and it's been a source of constant reference for me ever since I began my Ayurvedic journey five years ago, thanks to its continual updating. I thank them profusely for their generosity.

Note from the Institute: Guidelines provided in this table are general. Specific adjustments for individual requirements may need to be made, e.g. food allergies, strength of agni, season of the year and degree of dosha predominance or aggravation.

Key
* okay in moderation
** okay rarely

	Vata		Pitta		Kapha	
	Avoid	**Favour**	**Avoid**	**Favour**	**Avoid**	**Favour**
F R U I T S	Generally most dried fruit Apples (raw) Cranberries Dates (dry) Figs (dry) Pears Persimmons Pomegranates Prunes (dry) Raisins (dry) Watermelon	Generally most sweet fruit Apple purée (applesauce) Apples (cooked) Apricots Avocado Bananas Berries Cherries Coconut Dates (fresh) Figs (fresh) Grapefruit Grapes Kiwi fruit Lemons Limes Mangoes Melons Oranges Papaya Peaches Pineapple Plums Prunes (soaked) Raisins (soaked) Rhubarb Strawberries Tamarind	Generally most sour fruit Apples (sour) Apricots (sour) Bananas Berries (sour) Cherries (sour) Cranberries Grapefruit Grapes (green) Kiwi fruit** Lemons Mangoes (green) Oranges (sour) Peaches Persimmons Pineapple (sour) Plums (sour) Rhubarb Tamarind	Generally most sweet fruit Apple purée (applesauce) Apples (sweet) Apricots (sweet) Avocado Berries (sweet) Cherries (sweet) Coconut Dates Figs Grapes (black) Limes* Mangoes (ripe) Melons Oranges (sweet)* Papaya* Pears Pineapple (sweet)* Plums (sweet) Pomegranates Prunes Raisins Strawberries* Watermelon	Generally most sweet and sour fruit Avocado Bananas Coconut Dates Figs (fresh) Grapefruit Kiwi fruit Mangoes** Melons Oranges Papaya Pineapple Plums Rhubarb Tamarind Watermelon	Generally most astringent fruit Apple purée (applesauce) Apples Apricots Berries Cherries Cranberries Figs (dry)* Grapes* Lemons* Limes* Peaches* Pears Persimmons Pomegranates Prunes Raisins Strawberries*

	Vata		Pitta		Kapha	
	Avoid	**Favour**	**Avoid**	**Favour**	**Avoid**	**Favour**
VEGETABLES	Generally frozen, raw or dried vegetables	Generally vegetables should be cooked	Generally pungent vegetables	Generally sweet and bitter vegetables	Generally sweet and juicy vegetables	Generally most pungent and bitter vegetables
	Artichoke	Asparagus	Aubergine/ eggplant**	Artichoke	Courgettes (zucchini)	Artichoke
	Aubergine/ eggplant	Beetroot/beets	Beetroot/beets (raw)	Asparagus	Cucumber	Asparagus
	Beetroot tops/ beet greens**	Cabbage (cooked)*	Beetroot tops/ beet greens	Bean sprouts (not spicy)	Olives (black or green)	Aubergine/ eggplant
	Bitter melon	Carrots	Burdock root	Beetroot/beets (cooked)	Parsnips**	Beetroot/beets
	Broccoli	Cauliflower*	Courgettes/ zucchini	Bitter melon	Pumpkin	Beetroot tops/ beet greens
	Brussels sprouts	Coriander/ cilantro leaves	Daikon radish	Broccoli	Squash, summer	Bitter melon
	Burdock root	Courgettes/ zucchini	Garlic	Brussels sprouts	Sweet potatoes	Broccoli
	Cabbage (raw)	Cucumber	Green chillies	Cabbage	Taro root	Brussels sprouts
	Cauliflower (raw)	Daikon radish*	Horseradish	Carrots (cooked)	Tomatoes (raw)	Burdock root
	Celery	Fennel (anise)	Kohlrabi**	Carrots (raw)*		Cabbage
	Dandelion greens	Garlic	Leeks (raw)	Cauliflower		Carrots
	Horseradish**	Green beans	Mustard greens	Celery		Cauliflower
	Kale	Green chillies	Olives (green)	Coriander/ cilantro leaves		Celery
	Kohlrabi	Jerusalem artichoke*	Onions (raw)	Courgettes/ zucchini		Coriander/ cilantro leaves
	Mushrooms	Leafy greens*	Peppers (hot)	Cucumber		Daikon radish
	Olives (green)	Leeks	Prickly pear (fruit)	Dandelion greens		Dandelion greens
	Onions (raw)	Lettuce*	Radishes (raw)	Fennel (anise)		Fennel (anise)
	Peas (raw)	Mustard greens*	Spinach (cooked)**	Green beans		Garlic
	Peppers (sweet and hot)	Okra	Spinach (raw)	Jerusalem artichoke		Green beans
	Potatoes, white	Olives (black)	Sweet corn (fresh)**	Kale		Green chillies
	Prickly pear (fruit and leaves)	Onions (cooked)*	Tomatoes	Leafy greens		Horseradish
		Parsley*	Turnip tops/ turnip greens*			Jerusalem artichoke
		Parsnip				Kale

	Vata		Pitta		Kapha	
	Avoid	**Favour**	**Avoid**	**Favour**	**Avoid**	**Favour**
VEGETABLES (continued)	Squash (winter) Sweet corn (fresh)** Tomatoes (cooked)** Tomatoes (raw) Turnips Wheat grass sprouts	Peas (cooked) Pumpkin Radishes (cooked)* Spaghetti squash* Spinach (cooked)* Spinach (raw)* Sprouts* Squash, summer Swede/ rutabaga Sweet potatoes Taro root Turnip tops/ turnip greens* Watercress	Turnips Watercress	Leeks (cooked) Lettuce Mushrooms Okra Olives (black) Onions (cooked) Parsley Parsnips Peas Peppers (sweet) Potatoes Prickly pear (leaves) Pumpkin Radishes (cooked) Spaghetti squash Squash (winter and summer) Swede/ rutabaga Sweet potatoes Taro root Watercress* Wheat grass sprouts	Generally sweet and juicy vegetables Courgettes (zucchini) Cucumber Olives (black or green) Parsnips** Pumpkin Squash, summer Sweet potatoes Taro root Tomatoes (raw)	Kohlrabi Leafy greens Leeks Lettuce Mushrooms Mustard greens Okra Onions Parsley Peas Peppers (sweet and hot) Potatoes Prickly pear (fruit & leaves) Radishes Spaghetti squash* Spinach Sprouts Squash (winter) Swede/ rutabaga Sweet corn Tomatoes (cooked) Turnip tops/ turnip greens Turnips Watercress Wheat grass

	Vata		Pitta		Kapha	
	Avoid	**Favour**	**Avoid**	**Favour**	**Avoid**	**Favour**
G R A I N S	Barley Bread (with yeast) Buckwheat Cereals (cold, dry or puffed) Couscous Crackers Granola Maize/corn Millet Muesli Oat bran Oats (dry) Pasta** Polenta** Rice cakes** Rye Sago Spelt Tapioca Wheat bran	Amaranth* Durum flour Oats (cooked) Pancakes Quinoa Rice (all kinds) Seitan (wheat meat) Sprouted wheat bread (essene) Wheat	Bread (with yeast) Buckwheat Maize (corn) Millet Muesli** Oats (dry) Polenta** Rice (brown)** Rye	Amaranth Barley Cereal (dry) Couscous Crackers Durum flour Granola Oat bran Oats (cooked) Pancakes Pasta Quinoa Rice (basmati, white, wild) Rice cakes Seitan (wheat meat) Spelt Sprouted wheat bread (essene) Tapioca Wheat Wheat bran	Bread (with yeast) Oats (cooked) Pancakes Pasta** Rice (brown, white) Rice cakes** Wheat	Amaranth* Barley Buckwheat Cereal (cold, dry or puffed) Couscous Crackers Durum flour* Granola Maize/corn Millet Muesli Oat bran Oats (dry) Polenta Quinoa* Rice (basmati, wild)* Rye Seitan (wheat meat) Spelt* Sprouted wheat bread (essene) Tapioca Wheat bran

	Vata		Pitta		Kapha	
	Avoid	**Favour**	**Avoid**	**Favour**	**Avoid**	**Favour**
LEGUMES	Aduki beans Black beans Black-eyed peas Butter/lima beans Chickpeas Haricot/navy beans Kidney beans Lentils (brown) Miso** Peas (dried) Pinto beans Soya beans Soya flour Soya powder Split peas Tempeh White beans	Lentils (red)* Mung beans Mung dal Soy sauce* Soya cheese* Soya milk* Soya sausages* Tofu* Tur dal Urad dal	Miso Soy sauce Soya sausages Tur dal Urad dal	Aduki beans Black beans Black-eyed peas Butter/lima beans Chickpeas Haricot/navy beans Kidney beans Lentils (brown and red) Mung beans Mung dal Peas (dried) Pinto beans Soya beans Soya cheese Soya flour* Soya milk Soya powder* Split peas Tempeh Tofu White beans	Kidney beans Miso Soy powder Soy sauce Soya beans Soya cheese Soya flour Tofu (cold) Urad dal	Aduki beans Black beans Black-eyed peas Butter/lima beans Chickpeas Haricot/navy beans Lentils (red and brown) Mung beans* Mung dal* Peas (dried) Pinto beans Soya milk Soya sausages Split peas Tempeh Tofu (hot)* Tur dal White beans
DAIRY	Cow's milk (powdered) Goat's milk (powdered) Yogurt (natural, frozen or with fruit)	Most dairy is good! Butter Buttermilk Cheese (hard)* Cheese (soft) Cottage cheese Cow's milk Ghee Goat's cheese Goat's milk Ice cream* Sour cream* Yogurt (diluted and spiced)*	Butter (salted) Buttermilk Cheese (hard) Sour cream Yogurt (natural, frozen or with fruit)	Butter (unsalted) Cheese (soft, not aged, unsalted) Cottage cheese Cow's milk Ghee Goat's cheese (soft, unsalted) Goat's milk Ice cream Yogurt (freshly made and diluted)*	Butter (salted) Butter (unsalted)** Cheese (soft & hard) Cow's milk Ice cream Sour cream Yogurt (plain, frozen or with fruit)	Buttermilk* Cottage cheese (from skimmed/low-fat goat's milk) Ghee* Goat's cheese (unsalted and not aged)* Goat's milk (skimmed) Yogurt (diluted)

	Vata		Pitta		Kapha	
	Avoid	Favour	Avoid	Favour	Avoid	Favour
ANIMAL FOODS	Lamb Pork Rabbit Turkey (white) Venison	Beef Buffalo Chicken (dark) Chicken (white)* Duck Eggs Fish (freshwater or sea) Salmon Sardines Seafood Prawns/shrimp Tuna Turkey (dark)	Beef Chicken (dark) Duck Eggs (yolk) Fish (sea) Lamb Pork Salmon Sardines Seafood Tuna Turkey (dark)	Buffalo Chicken (white) Eggs (albumen or white only) Fish (freshwater) Rabbit Prawns/shrimp* Turkey (white) Venison	Beef Buffalo Chicken (dark) Duck Fish (sea) Lamb Pork Salmon Sardines Seafood Tuna Turkey (dark)	Chicken (white) Eggs Fish (freshwater) Prawns/shrimp Rabbit Turkey (white) Venison
CONDIMENTS	Chocolate Horseradish	Black pepper* Chutney, mango (sweet or spicy) Chilli peppers* Coriander/cilantro leaves* Dulse Gomasio Hijiki Kelp Ketchup Kombu Lemon Lime Lime pickle Mango pickle Mayonnaise Mustard Pickles Salt Seaweed Soy sauce Spring onions/scallions Sprouts* Tamari Vinegar	Chilli pepper Chocolate Chutney, mango (spicy) Gomasio Horseradish Kelp Ketchup Mustard Lemon Lime pickle Mango pickle Mayonnaise Pickles Salt (in excess) Soy sauce Spring onions/scallions Vinegar	Bean sprouts Black pepper* Chutney, mango (sweet) Coriander/cilantro leaves Dulse* Hijiki* Kombu* Lime* Salt* Seaweed* Tamari*	Chocolate Chutney, mango (sweet) Gomasio Kelp Ketchup** Lime Lime pickle Mango pickle Mayonnaise Pickles Salt Soy sauce Tamari Vinegar	Bean sprouts Black pepper Chilli peppers Chutney, mango (spicy) Coriander/cilantro leaves Dulse* Hijiki* Horseradish Lemon* Mustard (without vinegar) Seaweed* Spring onions/scallions

	Vata		Pitta		Kapha	
	Avoid	**Favour**	**Avoid**	**Favour**	**Avoid**	**Favour**
NUTS	None	In moderation: Almonds Black walnuts Brazil nuts Cashew nuts Charole Coconut Filberts Hazelnuts Macadamia nuts Peanuts Pecans Pine nuts Pistachios Walnuts	Almonds (with skin) Black walnuts Brazil nuts Cashew nuts Filberts Hazelnuts Macadamia nuts Peanuts Pecans Pine nuts Pistachios Walnuts	Almonds (soaked and peeled) Charole Coconut	Almonds (soaked and peeled)** Black walnuts Brazil nuts Cashew nuts Coconut Filberts Hazelnuts Macadamia nuts Peanuts Pecans Pine nuts Pistachios Walnuts	Charole
SEEDS	Popcorn Psyllium**	Chia Flax (linseed) Halva Pumpkin Sesame Sunflower Tahini	Chia Sesame Tahini	Flax (linseed) Halva Popcorn (no salt, buttered) Psyllium Pumpkin* Sunflower	Halva Psyllium** Sesame Tahini	Chia Flax* (linseed) Popcorn (no salt, no butter) Pumpkin* Sunflower*
OILS	Flaxseed	For internal and external use (most suitable at top of list): Sesame Ghee Olive Most other oils External use only: Coconut Avocado	Almond Apricot Corn Safflower Sesame	For internal and external use (most suitable at top of list): Sunflower Ghee Olive Rapeseed/ canola Soya Flaxseed Primrose Walnut External use only: Avocado Coconut	Apricot Avocado Coconut Flaxseed** Olive Primrose Safflower Sesame (internal) Soya Walnut	For internal and external use in small amounts (most suitable at top of list): Corn Rapeseed/ canola Sesame (external) Sunflower Ghee Almond

	Vata		Pitta		Kapha	
	Avoid	**Favour**	**Avoid**	**Favour**	**Avoid**	**Favour**
B E V E R A G E S	Alcohol (hard; red wine)	Alcohol (beer; white wine)*	Alcohol (hard; red and sweet wine)	Alcohol (beer; dry white wine)*	Alcohol (hard; beer; sweet wine)	Alcohol (dry wine, red or white)*
	Apple juice	Almond milk	Apple cider	Almond milk	Almond milk	Aloe vera juice
	Black tea	Aloe vera juice	Berry juice (sour)	Aloe vera juice	Caffeinated beverages**	Apple cider
	Caffeinated beverages	Apple cider	Caffeinated beverages	Apple juice	Carbonated drinks	Apple juice*
	Carbonated drinks	Apricot juice	Carbonated drinks	Apricot juice	Cherry juice (sour)	Apricot juice
	Chocolate milk	Berry juice (except for cranberry)	Carrot juice	Berry juice (sweet)	Chocolate milk	Berry juice
	Coffee	Carob*	Cherry juice (sour)	Black tea*	Coffee	Black tea (spiced)
	Cold dairy drinks	Carrot juice	Chocolate milk	Carob	Cold dairy drinks	Carob
	Cranberry juice	Chai (hot spiced milk)	Coffee	Chai (hot, spiced milk)*	Grapefruit juice	Carrot juice
	Iced tea	Cherry juice	Cranberry juice	Cherry juice (sweet)	Iced tea	Chai (hot, spiced milk)*
	Icy cold drinks	Grain 'coffee'	Grapefruit juice	Cool dairy drinks	Icy cold drinks	Cherry juice (sweet)
	Pear juice	Grape juice	Iced tea	Grain 'coffee'	Lemonade	Cranberry juice
	Pomegranate juice	Grapefruit juice	Icy cold drinks	Grape juice	Miso broth	Grain 'coffee'
	Prune juice**	Lemonade	Lemonade	Mango juice	Orange juice	Grape juice
	Soya milk (cold)	Mango juice	Papaya juice	Miso broth*	Papaya juice	Mango juice
	Tomato juice**	Miso broth	Pineapple juice	Mixed vegetable juice	Rice milk	Peach nectar
	V-8 juice	Orange juice	Sour juices	Orange juice*	Sour juices	Pear juice
		Papaya juice	Tomato juice	Peach nectar	Soya milk (cold)	Pineapple juice*
		Peach nectar	V-8 juice	Pear juice	Tomato juice	Pomegranate juice
		Pineapple juice		Pomegranate juice	V-8 juice	Prune juice
		Rice milk		Prune juice		Soya milk (hot and well spiced)
		Sour juices		Rice milk		
		Soya milk (hot and well spiced)*		Soya milk		
		Vegetable bouillon		Vegetable bouillon		

	Vata		Pitta		Kapha	
	Avoid	**Favour**	**Avoid**	**Favour**	**Avoid**	**Favour**
H E R B A L T E A S	Alfalfa**	Ajwan	Ajwan	Alfalfa	Liquorice**	Alfalfa
	Barley**	Bancha	Basil**	Bancha	Marshmallow	Bancha
	Basil**	Catnip*	Clove	Barley	Red zinger	Barley
	Blackberry	Chamomile	Eucalyptus	Blackberry	Rosehip**	Blackberry
	Borage**	Chicory*	Fenugreek	Borage		Burdock
	Burdock	Chrysanthe-	Ginger (dry)	Burdock		Chamomile
	Cinnamon**	mum*	Ginseng	Catnip		Chicory
	Cornsilk	Clove	Hawthorne	Chamomile		Cinnamon
	Dandelion	Comfrey	Juniper berry	Chicory		Clove
	Ginseng	Elderflower	Mormon tea	Comfrey		Comfrey*
	Hibiscus	Eucalyptus	Pennyroyal	Dandelion		Dandelion
	Hops**	Fennel	Red zinger	Fennel		Fennel*
	Jasmine**	Fenugreek	Rosehip**	Ginger (fresh)		Fenugreek
	Lemon balm**	Ginger (fresh)	Sage	Hibiscus		Ginger
	Mormon tea	Hawthorne	Sassafras	Hops		Ginseng*
	Nettle**	Juniper berry	Yerba mate	Jasmine		Hibiscus
	Passion	Kukicha*		Kukicha		Jasmine
	flower**	Lavender		Lavender		Juniper berry
	Red clover**	Lemongrass		Lemon balm		Kukicha
	Red zinger**	Liquorice		Lemongrass		Lavender
	Violet**	Marshmallow		Liquorice		Lemon balm
	Yarrow	Oat straw		Marshmallow		Lemongrass
	Yerba mate**	Orange peel		Nettle		Mormon tea
		Pennyroyal		Oat straw		Nettle
		Peppermint		Passion flower		Passion flower
		Raspberry*		Peppermint		Peppermint
		Rosehips		Raspberry		Raspberry
		Saffron		Red clover		Red clover
		Sage		Sarsaparilla		Sarsaparilla*
		Sarsaparilla		Spearmint		Sassafras
		Sassafras		Strawberry		Spearmint
		Spearmint		Violet		Strawberry
		Strawberry*		Wintergreen		Wintergreen
		Wintergreen*		Yarrow		Yarrow
						Yerba mate

	Vata		Pitta		Kapha	
	Avoid	**Favour**	**Avoid**	**Favour**	**Avoid**	**Favour**
S P I C E S		All spices are good Ajwan Allspice Almond extract Anise Asafoetida (hing) Basil Bay leaf Black pepper Caraway Cardamom Cayenne* Cinnamon Cloves Coriander seeds Cumin Dill Fennel Fenugreek* Garlic Ginger Marjoram Mint Mustard seeds Nutmeg Orange peel Oregano Paprika Parsley Peppermint Pippali Poppy seeds Rosemary Saffron Salt Savory Spearmint Star anise Tarragon Thyme Turmeric Vanilla Wintergreen	Ajwan Allspice Almond extract Anise Asafoetida (hing) Basil (dry) Bay leaf Cayenne Cloves Fenugreek Garlic Ginger (dry) Mace Marjoram Mustard seeds Nutmeg Oregano Paprika Pippali Poppy seeds Rosemary Sage Salt Savory Star anise Thyme	Basil (fresh) Black pepper* Caraway* Cardamom* Cinnamon Coriander seeds Cumin Dill Fennel Ginger (fresh) Mint Neem leaves* Orange peel* Parsley* Peppermint Saffron Spearmint Tarragon* Turmeric Vanilla* Wintergreen	Salt	All spices are good Ajwan Allspice Almond extract Anise Asafoetida (hing) Basil Bay leaf Black pepper Caraway Cardamom Cayenne Cinnamon Cloves Coriander seeds Cumin Dill Fennel* Fenugreek Garlic Ginger Marjoram Mint Mustard seeds Neem leaves Nutmeg Orange peel Oregano Paprika Parsley Peppermint Pippali Poppy seeds Rosemary Saffron Savory Spearmint Star anise Tarragon Thyme Turmeric Vanilla* Wintergreen

	Vata		Pitta		Kapha	
	Avoid	**Favour**	**Avoid**	**Favour**	**Avoid**	**Favour**
SWEETENERS	Maple syrup** White sugar	Barley malt Demerara/ turbinado Fructose Fruit juice concentrates Honey Jaggery Molasses Rice syrup Sugar cane juice, dried or fresh	White sugar** Honey** Jaggery Molasses	Barley malt Demerara/ turbinado Fructose Fruit juice concentrates Maple syrup Rice syrup Sugar cane juice, dried or fresh	Barley malt Demerara/ turbinado Fructose Jaggery Maple syrup Molasses Rice syrup Sugar cane juice, dried or fresh White sugar	Fruit juice concentrates Honey (raw and not processed)
FOOD SUPPLEMENTS	Barley green Brewer's yeast Vitamin K	Aloe vera juice* Amino acids Bee pollen Blue-green algae Royal jelly Spiralina Minerals: calcium, copper, iron, magnesium, zinc Vitamins: A, B_1, B_2, B_6, B_{12}, C, D, E, P (bioflavonoids) and folic acid	Amino acids Bee pollen** Royal jelly** Minerals: copper, iron Vitamins: B_2, B_6, C, E, P (bioflavonoids) and folic acid	Aloe vera juice Barley green Blue-green algae Brewer's yeast Spiralina Minerals: calcium, magnesium, zinc Vitamins: A, B_1, B_{12}, D and K	Minerals: potassium Vitamins: A, B_1, B_2, B_{12}, D and E	Aloe vera juice Amino acids Barley green Bee pollen Blue-green algae Brewer's yeast Royal jelly Spiralina Minerals: calcium, copper, iron, magnesium, zinc Vitamins: B_6, C, P (bioflavonoids) and folic acid

BODY-BALANCING RECIPES

First, Stock Your Larder

The Body Balance Diet is purposely designed to involve as little unfamiliar food as possible because I think it's important to eat food that's indigenous as well as food that's nutritious. But there are certain things I've recommended throughout this book, all of which I've gathered here for ease of creating shopping lists.

Herbs and Spices

The herbs and spices you may like to explore – many of which are included in the recipes at the back of this book – include:

Asafoetida: You may not have encountered this very pungent powder before – it's actually a natural gum resin (extracted from the tree) and imparts a very strong oniony flavour to food. It has an extremely strong odour, which will put many off, but if kept in an airtight container it shouldn't be too offensive.

The tiniest pinch can be added to curries – add at the start, straight to the heating oil or ghee – and once cooked, it imparts a rich, deep garlic/onion flavour to the food. It is particularly good in vegetarian curries – leafy green or pulse/bean varieties benefit from it, as it helps stimulate digestion (firing up agni), and reduce bloating and gas.

Black pepper: Please try to buy good quality organic black peppercorns and grind them yourself in a peppermill – the pepper strength will be far more effective than if you pick up a ready-ground mix. Pungent and heating, black pepper is fantastic for stimulating agni, and gets those all-important digestive juices flowing. Ideal for Kapha and Vata, it helps keep the digestive, respiratory and circulatory systems healthy. Not so great for Pitta, thanks to the heating properties, but a small grind is nevertheless still good for digestion, and when mixed with a cooling or oily base (ghee or coconut oil in particular) can still be enjoyed.

Cardamom: This is a real hero spice with multiple, important uses. Once of its main benefits is how effectively it shifts agni from the system – getting the gut to get rid of mucus and also helping to alkalize an acidic system. Ayurveda fans use it to dispel gas, reflux, bloating and even nausea (it's ideal for morning sickness, for example).

Ancient Egyptians chewed cardamom pods to help clean and brighten their teeth and freshen their breath. Digestion-boosting, and also aiding the body in the uptake of nutrients from food, it is very versatile as it can be used in both sweet and savoury dishes, and by all doshas.

Cinnamon: Organic ground cinnamon is a great store-cupboard staple. Both pungent and sweet, cinnamon has been proven to improve mood, soothe nervous tension and also strengthen the immune system. Its natural antiseptic properties, coupled with its ability to boost circulation, mean it's wonderful in the winter, as it's renowned for warming the internal system and shifting a build-up of Kapha. It's also a wonderful addition to food for those who have a sweet tooth – proven to stabilize blood sugar and satiate that pang for sweetness without any additional sugar needed.

Coriander/cilantro: Cooling and balancing (and good for all doshas), this can be used in three states – as leaves and stems, as a ground powder or as seeds – and all have their place. Rather a divisive herb (my Cypriot heritage meant I grew up eating the leaves raw in salads, which I adore), it does taste 'soapy' to some people, and this can be improved if you blend it, or macerate it into a paste (it's great in Thai-style curry pastes). I call coriander my 'palate cleanser' – the leaves, in particular, are invigorating and refreshing – great for shifting ama. It gets both body and mind balanced, and is also a potent natural immunity-booster.

Cumin: This spice is very, very important – considered by Indians to be the central spice (it's the second most commonly bought spice worldwide, after black pepper) – and has numerous benefits. For digestion, it is an ama-shifting godsend, as it's naturally very cleansing without being caustic or aggressive. It stimulates agni too – so you get cleansing and digestion-optimizing properties in one spice – as well as being great at getting overloaded livers back on track.

With its potent antibiotic properties, it's ideal if you're always run down and poorly, and its naturally comforting earthy warmth means it helps to create a great base for curries, stews and soups. Ground cumin is used most regularly, but cumin seeds are also valuable – and can be toasted and served on top of almost anything (they are particularly good on warm winter salads).

Ginger: Most cultures are familiar with ginger and use it in powder form in baked goods, and as fresh ginger, as in the classic honey-and-ginger tea. It's also recommended to those suffering morning or travel sickness, and it really can help. Its unique intense heat, sweetness and zest make it a wonderful digestion-boosting spice, but this heat also means it can shift Kapha, which is ideal in winter when we're all prone to chesty infections and mucous coughs. Naturally energizing, it is also healing, and can be used in dozens of ways – such as in soups and curries. Good for all doshas, but slightly less so for Pitta.

Saffron: A fabled spice, thanks to its expensive nature (it's harvested from the stamens of crocuses, which have a very low yield, meaning many thousands of flowers are grown to produce relatively meagre amounts of saffron). Recent research has suggested that saffron has anti-cancer properties, and Ayurvedically it does many things – helping to boost energy, digestion, mood and even sexual appetite. Many people waste the spice, though – it ought not to be added direct to food, but rather steeped in hot water (or added to stock at the start of cooking) until it releases all of its delicate aromatic spice and smoke.

Salt: the best salt you can use within an Ayurvedic diet is natural rock salt, and Himalayan pink rock salt is the queen of rock salts – very rich in body-supporting minerals and also linked to lower blood pressure.

Sweeteners

Ayurvedic recipes traditionally use the sugar cane derivative jaggery as a sweetener. As it's utterly unrefined it's a great sugar substitute and it has a lovely rich molasses-type flavour. I also use organic coconut-palm sugar and honey. Honey, however, should never be added to drinks when they are still very hot, or used in baking as its properties change when heated above 40°C/104°F.

Chyawanprash: A wonderful naturally sweet jam-like preserve that can be stirred into hot water to make a satisfying tri-doshic tea.

A Note on Measurements

I would say that very few of these recipes require you to be a stickler for exact measurements (apart, perhaps, from the bread).

Particularly with vegetables, add more or less of an ingredient if you so choose; it's your palate, and it's important to cook something 'your way' – which should come in time too, once you've worked out how you like your Ayurvedic food to be. As far as spices and herbs are concerned, though, I have endeavoured to offer the best possible balance within each recipe, so I'd advise that you don't go off-track here (not least because you might end up with something that's so over- or under-spiced that it's practically inedible). All veg listed in the ingredients are medium size unless stated otherwise.

A Note on Variations

The Taste Table is, as far as these recipes are concerned, still your oracle. I will often offer a couple of options and advise on which is best for which dosha, but if you're ever unsure, a quick glance at the Taste Table will clear up any doubt. For example, for my porridge options you can use your milk of choice, and I suggest goat's or rice milk; a look at the Taste Table will show that rice isn't ideal for Kapha, but warm soya is.

The Perfect Start: Brilliant Balancing Breakfasts

CARDAMOM CHIA SPICE PORRIDGE
Serves 1-2

Great for all seasons
Suits all dosha types

Oats seem to have been usurped by other 'pseudocereal' grains which are in fact complete plant proteins in disguise (quinoa, buckwheat, amaranth). Doubtless these all have wonderful nutritional qualities, but oats are pretty impressive too – cholesterol-reducing, blood-sugar stabilizing and also great at shifting a build-up of mucus within the gut.

They're yummy and good foods for both Vata and Pitta types, and oat bran is great for Kapha too. Pitta types should not eat an excessive amount of chia, so if you're planning to have this porridge regularly, swap in flaxseeds or sesame seeds every now and again.

200ml/scant 1 cup rice, goat or soya milk (consult
    Taste Table)
1 crushed cardamom pod
A pinch of cinnamon

A pinch of nutmeg
25g/generous ¼ cup rolled oats
25g/¼ cup fine oat bran
1 generous handful of chia seeds
Maple syrup or honey to sweeten

Pour the milk into a pan over a low heat, add the cardamom pod, cinnamon and nutmeg and stir to distribute evenly. Add the oats and oat bran to the pan and stir slowly over a medium heat until the mixture starts to thicken. Turn the heat to low and while the oats are cooking toast a handful of chia seeds (or buy them ready toasted) in a shallow frying pan, skillet or wok. Take the porridge off the heat when it's a thick and creamy texture and remove the cardamom pod. Sprinkle the toasted chia seeds on top and drizzle honey or maple syrup over the porridge before serving.

MILLET AND PERFECT PEAR PORRIDGE

Serves 1-2

Great for autumn and winter
Best for Kapha types

I had a version of this porridge on my retreat and it was hugely comforting, satisfying and delicious. It's one of just a few dishes that remain true to the Ayurvedic diet, even when not strictly following the rules – it blends fruit with grains, after all, but because the stewed, ripe fruit is so easily digested, as are the lighter milks and wheat-free millet, things break down at the same time, and don't cause digestive upset.

174

This porridge can be eaten by everyone at any time, but is particularly good during the colder, wetter months, and for Kapha types. It's also an ideal nourishing start to the day during your Ayurvedic immersion. If the pears are very soft, juicy and ripe there's actually no need to cook them, but otherwise they'll benefit from being popped into boiling water for a few minutes. Though I am not a fan of drinking goat's milk (it is, well, just a bit too 'goaty' for my tastes), it transforms into a very creamy rich loveliness when heated for porridge, which makes it ideal here. If, however, you're not keen, I'd recommend an unsweetened rice or coconut milk instead.

120ml/½ cup unsweetened rice or coconut milk
4 cardamom pods
1 small ripe pear, peeled
87g/½ cup cooked millet
1 handful of coconut flakes
Maple syrup or honey for sweetening (optional)

To cook the millet, use a ratio of 1 part millet to 2.5 parts water, simmering for 30–40 minutes, until tender. You could soak it overnight instead – in the same amount of water – then rinse and drain and add straight to the pan, bringing the mixture up to the boil, then only simmer for 10 minutes.

Pour the milk into a pan over a low heat, add the cardamom pods and stir to distribute evenly. If your pear is not yielding and soft, pop it into a separate pan of boiling water until a knife slips easily through the flesh, but not so long that it starts to disintegrate. Add your cooked millet to the pan now, stirring slowly and evenly, breaking up any clumps of millet as they form. Remove the pear from the boiling water and slice into delicate strips. Toast the coconut flakes in a shallow frying pan, skillet or wok. Check the porridge again – you want the mixture to be smooth and creamy. Turn the heat off once this has happened, then remove the cardamom pods and serve immediately with the thin slices of pear and a sprinkling of coconut flakes on top of the porridge. Add a drizzle of maple syrup or honey if you desire some extra sweetness.

WHOLESOME SPEEDY NUTTY BUTTER

Great for all seasons
Suits all dosha types

Ever since I started whizzing up my own nut butters I've not only saved myself money, but also the displeasure of eating less than truly delicious shop-bought peanut butter. If, like me, you love nut butter, spend just five minutes every few weeks making it for yourself and you'll never look back. Peanuts come bottom of the nut class in terms of mineral content, but I've whizzed up walnuts, cashews and almonds – separately and together, depending on what I fancy. Despite nuts not being my best foods (for either Pitta or Kapha), I've had no adverse reactions to my own nut butters. If you've always eaten a food and haven't suffered digestive upset or energy dips, then you've probably developed the ability to process it just fine, even if it isn't a dream food in Ayurvedic terms.

Around 300g/2 cups chopped nuts of your choosing (consult the
Taste Table)
Raw virgin coconut oil, at least 1 tbsp, but add to taste

If I'm going to eat nut butter more regularly, I'll stick with
peeled and soaked almonds, a dollop of raw virgin coconut oil,
and that's it – blend, blend, blend, adding more oil, until you
get the consistency you like, then spoon into a sterilized jar, and
it'll last for up to a month in a cool cupboard. Serve on toast,
alone, or with a drizzle of raw honey; on crackers with banana,
or even with savoury foods – it's lovely stirred through noodles
and served with tuna or chicken for a 'satay' taste.

SPELT SOLDIERS WITH COCONUT BUTTER AND HONEY

Great for all seasons
Suits Pitta and Kapha types
(use wholewheat toast for Vata)

Spelt bread is easy to make thanks to its high
gluten content, which means it doesn't need to
prove for as long as a traditional bread mixture.
If you don't want to bother making your own
bread, look for an organic spelt or rye loaf – or
at the very least, as unprocessed a loaf as you

177

can find. This great breakfast is only as 'great' as the bread!

Though I love coconut butter, I'd never considered using it for anything other than cookies and flapjacks until I started buying raw virgin coconut oil for cooking. It's one of the healthiest oils you can cook with, thanks to its naturally very high essential fatty acid content and shelf stability – it doesn't need to be hydrogenated to be made into an 'oil' – and its low oxidation level. One morning my curiosity got the better of me and I decided to swap my usual organic butter for this, on toast. It spreads beautifully, melting into the bread, and yes, you get that lovely cooling fresh coconut taste – it's subtle, but brilliant when served on steaming spelt toast and drizzled with raw honey or my wholesome speedy nutty butter.

Coconut oil does, however, increase Kapha, as it has a cooling effect. Given that it's such a wonder oil, I tell Kapha friends to go ahead and enjoy in meals where it really makes sense to use it (a coconut-based curry for example), but to stick to corn and rapeseed (canola) oil for most cooking.

GOAT'S CHEESE AND ARTICHOKE FLATBREADS

Makes 10 flatbreads with topping; serves 5

Great for spring and early summer
Suits all dosha types

Absolutely perfect for lazy weekend mornings when you don't want to be up at dawn, but fancy something brunch-like when you do surface. It's all in the simple, punchy flavour of the ingredients – the result is quick, easy and utterly delicious. It works so well because you have the gorgeous creamy acidity of the cheese alongside the sweet earthy softness of the artichokes, atop crusty, herby bread.

I prepare the artichoke hearts myself, by peeling them, cutting off the stems, then boiling them in lightly sea-salted water. I use the leaves as a snack (dipped into a lemony hummus), and use the hearts for cooking. If you can buy globe artichokes from a farmer's market or good deli when they're in season, this is ideal. You can use the preserved ones but they don't quite measure up in terms of flavour.

You can also buy pre-packaged flatbreads, but if you can spare the time to make these spelt and coriander/cilantro flatbreads, you won't regret it. Here's how:

Flatbreads
280g/2 cups spelt flour
3 tsp baking powder
A large pinch of Himalayan pink rock salt, or organic
    sea salt
1 bunch of coriander/cilantro leaves, chopped

179

2 tsp ground coriander
1 tsp ground cumin
280g/scant 1¼ cups Greek yogurt
Ghee, for cooking

Topping
10 small artichoke hearts
1 tbsp olive oil
A squeeze of fresh lemon
100g/3½ oz goat's cheese (just under 1 tbsp for
   each flatbread)
4 spring onions/scallions, sliced very finely
Sea salt and freshly ground black pepper

Mix the flour, baking powder, salt, coriander/cilantro, spices and yogurt in a bowl until everything is combined, then knead together for a couple of minutes until the dough becomes smooth and springy. Return the dough to the bowl and cover with cling film/plastic wrap and chill for an hour. When chilled, divide the dough into 10 pieces. Coat your work surface generously with spelt flour (occasionally I use semolina flour, which adds that 'pizza-like' grainy bottom to these flatbreads, which is pretty yummy too) and roll each piece out until it's an even thickness of 2–3mm/¹⁄₁₆–⅛in.

To cook the flatbreads on a pizza stone (a special stone you place in the oven at its highest setting to absorb heat, which then cooks your dough at a higher temperature, faster – mimicking a pizza oven) place your flatbreads directly onto the preheated stone in the oven and let them cook until they start to puff up (you should see lovely aerated sections bubbling up), around a minute on each side if the stone is really hot.

To cook the flatbreads in a pan, you'll need a non-stick one that's large and flat enough for the bread. Heat the pan on the stove until it's smoking, add some ghee, then fling the bread straight on to it, and flip after a minute or two.

Once your flatbreads are ready, you can get your topping ready in seconds. I like to pan-fry my artichoke hearts in olive oil to warm them through and add a slightly nuttier roasted flavour by searing some of the edges. I then remove them when piping hot, squeeze on some lemon juice, cut into thin slices and place onto the flatbread with a generous smudge of goat's cheese, some razor-thin sprinkles of spring onion/scallion, a hearty grind of black pepper and a wee pinch of sea salt. Eat immediately!

Beautifully Balancing (and Satisfying) Lunches

Eating a larger meal in the middle of the day is in keeping with Ayurvedic principles – you'll digest it far more effectively than at other times because agni is strongest in the middle of the day, and you will also set yourself up to have stable blood sugar levels throughout the late afternoon (skipping those sugary office snacks) and feel less hungry once dinnertime rolls around (when a lighter meal will be just the ticket). Eating three courses for lunch is often encouraged on Ayurvedic immersions (every day of mine I was presented with a light seasonal salad starter, a delicious wholesome warm main meal and an Ayurvedic 'dessert' – a nut or grain porridge, a light fresh mint sorbet, a coconut crème mousse). If you have the time at weekends, try to get into the habit of a more substantial lunch and a much lighter dinner. I know it's harder to do during the working week, when lunchbreaks seem to be getting shorter and shorter and most of us barely have the time to wolf down a single sandwich, but if the opportunity for a proper out-of-office lunch presents itself, try to take it. Or take advantage of the communal work kitchen/canteen/local park bench to sit and eat at a calmer pace in a more enjoyable way.

CAULIFLOWER AND LENTIL CURRY
Serves 4

Great for spring, autumn and winter
Suits all dosha types; Pitta types should leave out the
spinach or substitute it with a seasonal cabbage or kale

A delicious filling curry that is mildly spiced but packed with flavour.

3 tbsp olive oil
1 medium-sized cauliflower, cut into 2cm/¾in pieces
2 garlic cloves, finely chopped
1 large onion, peeled and finely chopped
1 tbsp black mustard seeds
1 tbsp ground coriander
½ tbsp tamarind paste (for Vata only)

2 tbsp sun-dried tomato purée paste

1 tsp mild chilli powder

2 tsp garam masala

800g/3½ cups canned chopped tomatoes

180ml/½ cup hot vegetable stock (preferably
   homemade)

150g/¾ cup dry red lentils

3 big handfuls (approx 100g/3½ oz) raw spinach,
   or kale for Pitta types

1 handful coriander/cilantro leaves, roughly chopped

Heat 2 tablespoons of the olive oil in a large heavy-bottomed pan, and fry the cauliflower until lightly roasted and golden. Remove the cauliflower from the pan and leave to one side. Heat the remaining oil in the same pan and fry the garlic and onions for 5–6 minutes until yielding, transparent and soft. Add the mustard seeds until they begin to pop and release their aroma, then the other spices (except the coriander/cilantro leaves) and pastes and warm through, for 2–3 minutes. Add the canned tomatoes, hot vegetable stock, lentils and spinach or kale, and put the cauliflower back into the pan. Bring it all to a steady boil, then lower the heat until the mixture is simmering. Partly cover, and continue to simmer for 25 minutes. Once the vegetables are all tender and the lentils soft and swollen, remove from the heat. Finish with the coriander and serve.

TRI-DOSHIC TAZE FASULYE
Serves 4–6

Great for summer
Suits all dosha types

This green bean stew is my favourite Turkish meal. Every time I visit my mother's house I ask her to make this, and everyone in my family cooks it their own way (my father uses a pinch of cinnamon; my mother makes it spicy with lots of chilli flakes) – I make it with added Ayurvedic spicing and succulent chicken, and serve it with basmati rice, which is suitable for all doshas.

If you're able to get your hands on fresh seasonal green beans (which in the UK are picked young in early summer and retain a delicious sweetness) this will taste so much better, although I've often used frozen organic green beans which are 'field-to-frozen', so that they retain their goodness. If you're vegetarian this is just as delicious with the meat left out, but I really do enjoy it with the juicy chicken and it makes the meal more filling too. The 'white meat' of the chicken is tri-doshic (i.e. it suits all three doshas), but darker meat is only recommended for Vata. Although I often use thigh meat myself in other recipes, I tend to use thick strips of breast for this as they do not dry out when poached slowly, as they are in this stew.

1 medium onion, finely chopped
4 garlic cloves, finely chopped
½ tsp ground ginger
½ tsp ground cumin
½ tsp ground coriander

3 tbsp olive oil

2 large chicken breasts, cut into 2.5cm/1in thick strips

500g/1lb 2oz fine green beans, topped, tailed,
    trimmed and cut into 4cm/1½in pieces

400g/1¾ cups canned chopped tomatoes

125ml/½ cup water

A pinch of coconut sugar

Sea salt and freshly ground black pepper

Start by sautéing the onion, garlic and spices, with a pinch of salt, in the olive oil – you don't want to brown the onion and garlic, but to soften and sweeten them instead. When they are soft, add the strips of chicken and toss these in the oils and spices until most of the chicken has coloured and started to cook. Then add the green beans and canned tomatoes and cook for 3–4 minutes, to warm everything through. Pour the water into the pot (the beans cook down so it's fine if they're not completely submerged), and add a pinch of coconut sugar, then season with salt and black pepper and bring to the boil. Turn the heat down, put the lid on and simmer for 35–45 minutes (if the beans are frozen you may need the longer time, if fresh, less time) until the beans are very soft and tender – a knife-point should slip through them easily. Remove from the heat and let it cool slightly before serving with rice.

SPRING VEG AND TROUT SCRUMBLE

Serves 4

Great for spring and early summer
(also works for any season with adapted seasonal veg)
Suits all dosha types, with less garlic for Pitta

I made this by accident one spring while attempting to make a Spanish-omelette-type 'tortilla', and liked it so much I now make it every couple of weeks. The recipe can be adapted to suit any type of seasonal veg – I use spring vegetables here (spring onions/scallions, capsicum peppers, peas and wild garlic) – but in summer it's delicious with courgettes/zucchini, and in autumn with finely chopped squash and white goat's cheese. This is also lovely with salmon (which is good for Vata) – but as salmon is not advised for Pitta or Kapha, I've used freshwater trout (freshwater fish is better for both Pitta and Kapha).

I've used egg whites here as they are tri-doshic, but Vata and Kapha types can happily use the whole egg (I am Pitta, and often do too – knowing that egg yolks might not be ideal, but that their rich nutritional value is not to be missed out on too often).

1 large wild trout fillet steak (approx 170g/6oz)
1 lime, half cut into wedges, half squeezed for juice
2 tbsp olive oil (not virgin)
6 spring onions/scallions, finely chopped
2 yellow or orange capsicum peppers
80g/generous ½ cup frozen peas
6 large leaves of wild garlic, washed and cut into
    thin slivers
A large pinch of Himalayan pink rock salt

5 egg whites, whisked
Fresh basil, finely chopped, to taste
Freshly ground black pepper

Preheat the oven to 200°C/400°F/gas mark 6.

Grind some black pepper over the trout fillet then place onto a sheet of foil with a wedge of lime and make a parcel, ensuring you've sealed all the gaps. Pop it into the oven and bake for 15 minutes. Warm the oil in a pan, then add the spring onions/scallions, peppers, peas and wild garlic, with the salt and a grinding of black pepper. Cook on low heat for 10 minutes, softening the peppers and spring onions and ensuring the peas are cooked and warmed through. Remove the fish from the oven and check it's cooked through. Break up into chunky flakes and add to the pan. Once you're happy with the veg, pour the eggs over the mixture and stir through gently until you get nice clumps of veg, egg and fish. Toss the basil onto the food and give it one last stir through. Turn off the heat and sprinkle some lime juice over the mix, then serve.

TECHNICOLOUR TURKEY AND WILD RICE SALAD

Serves 2

Great for spring, summer and early autumn
Suits Pitta and Kapha types, but Kapha should leave out
olives, and substitute carrot for courgette/zucchini

This is one of those meals I crave if I've had a too-busy week, am over-hungry and under-nourished. It's a pretty simple salad, but a very balanced and filling one, and a few easy adjustments make it suitable for all doshas.

I like to heat all the vegetables through in a pan so that they're slightly cooked before I assemble the salad, as it makes it far more digestible and also means you can eat it in spring and autumn, as it's still warming.

1 large turkey steak

2 large sticks of celery, washed, trimmed and diced

Pitta: 1 medium-sized courgette/zucchini, peeled and grated; Kapha: 1 large carrot, peeled and grated

3 small spring onions/scallions, washed, trimmed and finely chopped

Approx 300g/1⅔ cups cooked and drained white beans (I like cannellini, but haricot/navy or butter/lima beans also work well)

80g/½ cup cooked wild rice

Freshly ground black pepper

A squeeze of lime

Olive or coconut oil for frying and to serve

1 large handful of good black olives, to serve

Preheat the oven to 220°C/425°F/gas mark 7. Turkey can easily dry out, so get an oven-safe frying pan nice and hot on the stove first, then quickly brown the turkey steak on both sides in olive or coconut oil to seal it and keep juices in. Then pop the pan into the oven for 5–6 minutes to finish cooking it through. Add some more olive oil, the celery, courgette/zucchini or carrot, and spring onions/scallions to the pan and heat all the veg through – until they're yielding slightly, but still with nice crunch. Then add the beans and the rice, with a good grinding of black pepper.

When everything is nice and warm, remove from the heat and serve with the turkey from the oven, sliced into thin strips on top, a good glug of virgin olive oil, and garnish with the olives and squeeze of lime to finish.

TECHNICOLOUR TUNA SALAD

Serves 2

Great for autumn and winter
Suits Vata types

This is a version of the recipe above to make it suitable for Vata. The ingredients are a tad different, but everything else is prepared and assembled in the same way.

1 small fresh beetroot/beet
1 small sweet potato
1 sprig of fresh thyme
1 large tuna steak
1 tbsp virgin olive oil
3 small spring onions/scallions, washed, trimmed
   and finely chopped
1 large handful of black olives
164g/1 cup cooked wild rice
A squeeze of fresh lime
Freshly ground black pepper

189

Preheat the oven to 190°C/375°F/gas mark 5. Wash the beetroot/ beet and sweet potato, then cut off the rough ends and any leaves, but leave the skins on and wrap in foil with a sprig of fresh thyme. Roast for an hour until both are soft and tender. When the veg is cool enough to handle, peel the skins off both, and dice the flesh of the beetroot/beet and sweet potato. Sear the tuna steak in a hot non-stick pan for 1–2 minutes on each side, until browned, but leave the middle pink. Remove and slice the fish into thin strips. Put the olive oil and spring onions/scallions in the pan that held the tuna, and lightly sauté with the roasted thyme, olives and wild rice. Mix in the roasted veg, toss together with a squeeze of lime and a generous grinding of black pepper and serve.

BASMATI RICE AND CHARRED VEGETABLE SALAD

Serves 2–4 (4 as a starter or 2 as a main course)

Great for spring and early summer
Suits all dosha types

A *warm vegetarian salad that you'll make again and again.*

200g/1¼ cups just-cooked basmati rice
3 tbsp extra virgin olive oil
1 red capsicum pepper, chopped
1 yellow capsicum pepper, chopped
3 spring onions/scallions, chopped
1 courgette/zucchini, sliced into thin cross-sections
¼ small butternut or cochina squash, sliced into
    thin cross-sections

2 garlic cloves
1 tsp fresh goat's cheese, crumbled
1 handful of fresh mint leaves, shredded
Juice of 1 small lemon
Sea salt and freshly ground black pepper
Sumac, for sprinkling

Stir in a good drizzle of the olive oil and cover the cooked rice until fully cooled. Heat a griddle, frying pan or skillet, toss on the vegetables and cook until they begin to char visibly. Add the charred vegetables to the rice. Crush or grate the garlic and add to the bowl. Sprinkle over a teaspoon or so of crumbled goat's cheese (this is intended as a seasoning so only a small amount is needed) and the mint leaves. Stir through with the remaining olive oil, the lemon juice, and salt and pepper to taste. Top with a generous sprinkling of sumac and serve.

SQUASH AND RED LENTIL TAGINE WITH FLAX DRESSING

Serves 4

Great for late autumn and all winter
Great for all dosha types

A really healing and nourishing meal which is nicely substantial but doesn't overtax the stomach. With its earthy balanced spicing it is ideal for warming up in the colder months and the iron boost from the chlorophyll-rich kale gives ailing immune systems a helping hand too.

1 tbsp olive oil

A large pinch of hot red chilli flakes (use sweet or mild chilli for Pitta)

1 red onion, roughly chopped

300g/10½ oz peeled butternut or coquina squash, roughly cubed

1 small courgette/zucchini, roughly cubed

1 tbsp sun-dried tomato purée paste or ordinary tomato purée paste

2 tsp paprika

2 tsp ground coriander

2 tsp grated nutmeg

500ml/2¼ cups vegetable stock

80g/½ cup red lentils

2 handfuls of shredded cavolo nero/Tuscan kale or any winter cabbage

Sea salt and freshly ground black pepper

1 handful of toasted pine nuts, to scatter

1 handful of flat-leaf parsley, chopped, to scatter

Quinoa, to serve

Flax dressing

1 tbsp flaxseed oil

A drizzle of extra virgin olive oil

A squeeze of lemon juice

A pinch of Himalayan pink rock salt

Heat the olive oil in a saucepan or tagine and add the hot red chilli flakes. Add the onion and the cubes of squash and courgette/zucchini. When the onion begins to sizzle, add the tomato paste and stir together. Add the paprika, coriander and nutmeg. Pour over the vegetable stock and stir in the red lentils. Grind in a small amount of salt and pepper at this point. Bring the tagine close to the boil before turning the heat right down.

If using a saucepan, partially cover to allow some of the steam to condense back into the pan. Simmer for around an hour or until the tagine thickens and the edges of the squash begin to fall away. This will help to thicken and sweeten the dish. At the end of cooking add the cavolo nero/Tuscan kale and simmer for a further 5 minutes before removing from the heat. Taste and season as needed with sea salt and black pepper.

Mix all the ingredients for the dressing together in a small bowl. Serve on quinoa and scatter each serving with toasted pine nuts, a good drizzle of the dressing and chopped flat-leaf parsley.

Divine (Easily Digested) Dinners

One-Pot Wonders

I mentioned earlier in the book that one-pot wonders are a truly Ayurvedic inspiration – according to Ayurveda you can cook competing/contradicting foods in a single pot and the differences will disappear in the process. It's a great way to occasionally do away with food-combining rules and offer up a bit more foodie freedom. I love these one-pot wonders for dinner because they're very easily digested, nourishing, satisfying and a great healing meal at the end of a hard day.

SOUL-SOOTHING STEW

Serves 6 (or makes 6 portions, ideal for your three-day immersion diet)

Great for all seasons
Suits all dosha types

This simple stew, based on traditional Ayurvedic kitchari, is designed to tax the body as little as possible and help it expel ama. It suits every dosha and also provides lots of nourishment as it contains a lovely balance of both protein and carbohydrate. The mung dal and mung beans both need to be soaked overnight to ensure this meal taxes the digestive system as little as possible when eaten. Soak in clean, filtered water and if you're going to cook the meal the next night or afternoon, drain and rinse the beans in the morning, then put them back into clean water until you're ready to cook them.

You can play around with several dosha-specific additions to this, which will also add interest if you're eating it several times over the course of your immersion. Adding seasonal dosha-specific vegetables into the pot at the last stage is ideal. Be creative – you can easily use sweet potato, courgette/zucchini, greens, capsicum peppers . . . It's also lovely served with dosha-specific accompaniments – a squeeze of lime, desiccated/dry unsweetened coconut, a dollop of coconut cream, fresh chilli, coriander/ cilantro. Be imaginative and experiment, and you'll enjoy your stew all the more.

185g/1 cup basmati rice
90g/½ cup mung dal (also called split yellow peas/
    lentils), soaked overnight
100g/½ cup dry green mung beans, soaked overnight
3 tsp ghee, but Pitta and Kapha can use coconut oil
1 tsp ground turmeric
2 tsp cumin seeds
1 tbsp fennel seeds
1 tbsp mustard seeds
½ tsp ground coriander
1cm/½in piece of fresh ginger, chopped and grated
Himalayan pink rock salt and freshly ground
    black pepper

Rinse the rice, mung dal and soaked beans together in a sieve. Drain, then leave to one side. Heat your ghee or coconut oil in a large heavy-bottomed pan. Once it is melted, add the turmeric, cumin and fennel seeds. Let the spices heat through in the oil until they release their full aroma. Then add the rice, beans and dal to the pan, stirring everything through. When the rice and beans start to release their starch and become a little sticky, add the rest of your spices – mustard seed, ground coriander and fresh ginger, along with the salt and black pepper. Half fill the pan with filtered water (4–6cm/1½–2½in above the beans and rice), give everything a good stir and bring to the boil, then pop the lid on and let it simmer away for 20–25 minutes, until the beans and rice are completely soft and tender (al dente rice has no place here – this is about easy-as-possible digestion, remember).

GOLDEN CARROT SOUP

Serves 4–6 (6 as a starter or 4 as a main course)

Great for all seasons
Suits Vata and Pitta types

The earthy sweet butteriness of this soup is intensely comforting and nourishing – and it's always nice to remind yourself that butter is not a bad food. It's best to use ghee, but fine to use butter on occasion. For a heartier lunch serve with a lovely wedge of spelt or rye bread, with my hummus, one of my 'pesto' sauces or a homemade olive tapenade (simply whizz up 100g/½ cup of pitted and chopped olives in a food processor and add black pepper). It's also a great one to make in advance and freeze as it tastes just as fresh upon reheating.

½ tsp saffron
1 litre/4½ cups vegetable stock
2 tbsp ghee or unsalted butter
1 tsp Himalayan pink salt
2 generous pinches ground black pepper
½ tsp fennel seeds
2 large golden onions, peeled and diced
1 garlic clove (or 2 'young' garlic cloves), peeled and
   crushed/minced
4 carrots, peeled and diced
1 bay leaf (Pitta should leave this out)
1 tbsp fresh parsley, finely chopped
Virgin olive oil, for drizzling

In a heatproof bowl, add the saffron to the hot vegetable stock and leave for 30 minutes. Melt the ghee in a large pan, then add a pinch of the salt and a pinch of the pepper, together with the fennel seeds, the onions, garlic and carrots, and sauté over a medium heat for a couple of minutes until the fennel seeds give off their aroma and the vegetables start to soften. Add the bay leaf (if using) and half the parsley and continue to sauté for 5 minutes. Add the saffron and vegetable stock, with the remaining salt and pepper, and stir well. Bring to a gentle boil, then replace lid and let simmer until everything is meltingly tender, around 20 minutes. Transfer to a blender (or use a hand blender in the existing pan), and blend to your desired consistency. Serve with the remaining parsley and a drizzle of olive oil on top.

ROOT TO CARROT-TOP SOUP

Serves 4–6 (6 as a starter or 4 as a main course)

Great for spring to early summer
Suits Vata and Kapha types

With carrots, potatoes, spring greens/collard greens and sunflower seeds, this is a life-affirming soul-warming bowl of food, and wonderful during the crisper spring months. Spring greens are packed with flavour and alkalizing nutrients, and you can also use whatever you find locally – Savoy cabbage, mustard greens, Swiss chard – it's your call.

Use new potatoes (varieties differ greatly from country to country and region to region – simply try to buy the freshest organic new potatoes that you can), but small salad potatoes work well here too. Much of the flavour of this soup comes from the roasted garlic, *so ensure your garlic is as fresh and potent as possible (cloves that have been sitting around in the back of the refrigerator or at the bottom of the veg drawer for several months will not suffice!).*

1 medium head of garlic, halved
Olive oil, for roasting
1 tbsp ghee
2 large onions, peeled and diced
½ piece of ginger, peeled and crushed/minced
1 tsp sea salt
6 new potatoes (Vata should use yam or sweet
    potato), washed and diced
4 carrots, peeled and diced
450g/1lb spring greens/collard greens, shredded
1 tsp ground cumin
½ tsp ground cinnamon
1 handful of raw sunflower seeds, shelled (you'll need
    around 15 per serving)

Preheat the oven to 190°C/375°F/gas mark 5. Brush the two halves of the head of garlic with olive oil and roast in the oven until the garlic in the skins is butter-soft – this will take around an hour. Squeeze the cloves out of their skins when they are cool enough to handle. Heat the ghee in a large pan, then add the onions and ginger, a pinch of the salt, and sauté until they begin to soften. Add the roasted garlic, potatoes and spring greens/collard greens, and sauté for several minutes, then add the cumin and cinnamon and continue to cook until all the veg starts to soften. Pour in enough filtered water to cover the veg, add the remaining salt, put the lid on and bring to the boil. Reduce the heat and allow to simmer until the vegetables are tender. Serve the soup as it is, with soft chunks of veg, or blend to a smoother, thicker consistency – it's great both ways. Sprinkle the raw shelled sunflower seeds on top to serve.

RED LENTIL AND COCONUT SOUP

Serves 4

Great for spring and summer
Suits all dosha types

A *hearty soup that is also wonderfully cooling thanks to the natural Pitta-dousing effects of the herbs, vegetables and coconut milk used. Served with a small wedge of rye or spelt bread (Vata types can have wheat as long as they don't have an intolerance) or a light spelt chapatti, this is a good balanced dinner.*

Vata can add some sweet potato or squash to the soup for extra calories and sweet carbohydrate which they thrive on, and also use extra ghee during cooking; Pitta should sprinkle the soup with chopped coriander/cilantro leaves for extra cooling effect; and Kapha should add a pinch of chilli to the herb mix.

200g/1 cup dry red lentils
960ml/scant 4 cups filtered water
1 thumb-sized piece of fresh ginger, very
    finely chopped
2 tsp ground coriander
1 tsp ground turmeric
A small pinch of asafoetida

1 tbsp ghee
1 leek, chopped
2 tsp cumin seeds
½ tsp sea salt
1 tsp garam masala
¼ tsp ground cinnamon
A generous drizzle of coconut milk, to serve
4 lime wedges, to serve

Rinse the lentils well and ensure there are no stones in them. Small red lentils do not usually need to be soaked overnight, but do check the packet of the lentils you're using as some varieties will differ. Pour the lentils into a large saucepan with a heavy bottom, add the water and bring it up to the boil. When cooking lentils you often get a brown/grey foam (scurf) that builds on the top – skim it off with a wooden spoon and discard. Add the fresh ginger, ground coriander, turmeric and asafoetida. Reduce the heat and let it simmer for 45 minutes with the lid on. In a separate frying pan or skillet, heat up the ghee, then sauté the leek and cumin seeds. You want them to colour slightly, so keep on a low heat and make sure they don't burn.

Add these sautéed ingredients to the pan with the cooking lentils. Now add your salt, garam masala and cinnamon. Give everything a good stir to ensure it's all evenly cooked and spiced. You can choose to blend it in the pan to create a super-smooth and thick lentil soup, or leave it as it is, with a bit of texture from the lentils and leeks to add interest. Serve with a generous drizzle of coconut milk, and a wedge of lime to squeeze onto the soup just before eating.

LOVE BROTH

Serves 4

Great for all seasons
Suits all dosha types

This lovely fragrant, fresh but satisfying soup seemingly puts the world to rights. Whenever I curl up with a bowl I know I'll feel better for it, which is why it's great for anyone on the immersion (a culinary cuddle, if you will).

1 tbsp ghee
1 tbsp olive oil
2 large white onions, peeled and diced
2 large garlic cloves (1 small clove for Pitta), crushed/minced
1 tsp turmeric
1 tsp Himalayan pink rock salt
1 tsp ground black pepper
1 large bunch of leafy seasonal greens (any combination of pak choi, collard greens, Swiss chard, lettuce), finely chopped
2.5cm/1in piece of fresh ginger, finely minced
Approx 15g/1 cup coriander/cilantro leaves, chopped
120ml/½ cup coconut milk
A squeeze of lime (optional)

Over a low heat, warm the ghee and/or olive oil in a heavy-bottomed pot and sauté the onions and garlic, with the turmeric, salt and pepper. After a minute add the greens and ginger, and coat with the oil and spice. Keep on a low heat, par-cooking the

201

vegetables for a few minutes, until they begin to soften. Top up with water until it's 5cm/2in above the vegetables. Simmer on a low heat for 30 minutes, or until all the vegetables are buttery-soft – add most of the coconut milk now (saving a drizzle for later), stir into the soup, and leave for another minute, then turn off the heat. Serve with the coriander/cilantro leaves and, if you desire, an additional drizzle of coconut milk and a squeeze of lime.

CHICKPEA AND KALE CURRY WITH SPELT CHAPATTIS
Serves 2 generously

Great for spring and early winter
Suits all dosha types

2 garlic cloves, finely chopped
1 thumb-sized piece of fresh ginger
1 tbsp extra virgin coconut oil
1 tsp cumin seeds
1 tsp mustard seeds
A pinch of fennel seeds
1 small onion, finely chopped or grated
2 fresh chillies, finely chopped
400g/2½ cups cooked or canned chickpeas
1 tsp ground coriander
¾ tsp ground turmeric
1 tsp paprika
3 tomatoes, chopped
1 large handful of shredded kale
1 handful of coriander/cilantro, chopped

A squeeze of lime
Sea salt and freshly ground black pepper

Chapattis
A drizzle of ground nut oil or rapeseed/canola oil
A pinch of sea salt
140g/1 cup wholemeal spelt flour, plus extra for rolling

Make a paste with the garlic, ginger and a drizzle of water in a mortar or food processor. Heat the extra virgin coconut oil in a saucepan. Add the cumin seeds, mustard seeds and fennel seeds and cook until they begin to pop. Add the garlic and ginger paste, onion and chillies and stir. Add the chickpeas and ground coriander, turmeric and paprika, a good pinch of sea salt and black pepper. Add in the tomatoes, stirring for 1 minute, then pour in 150ml/²⁄₃ cup water. Reduce the heat and allow to simmer for 15–20 minutes, adding a little water if the curry becomes too thick. Add the kale and simmer for a further 5 minutes. Taste and add salt and pepper as required. Finish with the coriander/cilantro and a squeeze of lime juice.

To make the chapattis, add the oil and salt to the flour. Add water sparingly as you go, drizzle by drizzle, blending it with the flour until a firm dough (not runny or wet) is formed. Knead for a minute or two. Divide the dough into golf-ball-sized pieces, flour a work surface and roll each ball into a very thin disc. Heat a dry frying pan or skillet on the stove and cook the chapattis one at a time, for a minute or two on each side. Remove them when cooked through, browned and puffed, and stack and cover with a clean tea/dish towel to keep them warm. Serve warm with the curry.

DEEP AND YUMMY COCOA-SPICE CHILLI

Serves 2 generously

Great for autumn and winter

Ideal for Vata types; Pitta and Kapha can enjoy occasionally

2 tbsp olive oil, plus extra for drizzling

1½ tsp cumin seeds

A large pinch of red chilli flakes

3 garlic cloves, finely chopped or crushed

1 medium red onion, chopped

1 red capsicum pepper, chopped

1 tbsp sun-dried tomato purée paste or normal
   tomato purée paste

400g/1¾ cups canned chopped tomatoes

125ml/½ cup red wine

400g/2 cups red lentils

1½ tsp ground coriander

2 tsp dried oregano

2 tsp paprika

1 tsp raw cocoa powder

Juice of 1 lime

1 handful of coriander/cilantro, chopped

Sea salt and freshly ground black pepper

Saffron basmati rice or corn tortillas, to serve

Heat the olive oil in a saucepan. Add the cumin seeds and cook until they begin to pop, then put in the red chilli flakes. Add the garlic and the onion and cook for 1 minute. Add the red pepper and stir in the tomato purée paste. Pour in the canned tomatoes and the red wine. Add the lentils and ground coriander, oregano, paprika and cocoa powder. Add a good pinch of sea salt and good grind of black pepper. Reduce the heat and allow to simmer for 1 hour. Taste and season further if required. Finish with the lime juice, a drizzle of extra virgin olive oil and the coriander/cilantro. Serve with saffron basmati rice or corn tortillas for tacos.

Nourishing, Savoury Snacks

MY HUMMUS
Serves 6

Great for all seasons
Suits Pitta and Kapha types

160g/1 cup cooked or canned chickpeas
2 cloves garlic, crushed/minced (use a press for
   fine pulp)
2 tbsp tahini
1 tsp cumin seed powder
1 tsp organic sea salt
3 tbsp extra virgin olive oil
Juice of 1 lime
A small pinch of Asafoetida

Put everything into the food processer and whizz up to your desired consistency. I like to scatter fresh-cut coriander leaves/ cilantro and cooked chickpeas over the top, drizzle some extra virgin oil over it, adding a squeeze of lime and a pinch of paprika before serving.

SWEET POTATO AND RED LENTIL DIP

Serves 6

Great for summer and autumn
Suits Vata and Pitta types

This can be perfect served with steamed vegetables, pitta wedges or chapattis, or even as a brilliant filling for a sandwich – try it with roasted seasonal vegetables (courgette/zucchini, onion, capsicum peppers) or the lovely crunchy-fresh coleslaw below.

1 medium sweet potato, peeled and diced
2 garlic cloves, bashed/crushed
3 tbsp extra virgin olive oil
300g/1½ cups red lentils
60ml/¼ cup fresh lime juice (approx 2 limes)
½ tsp Himalayan pink rock salt
½ tsp freshly ground black pepper
1 handful of coriander/cilantro, very finely chopped

Preheat the oven to 200°C/400°F/gas mark 6. Roast the sweet potato and garlic cloves (in skins), with a drizzle of the olive oil, in the oven for 15–20 minutes, until both are soft and slightly caramelized. While you're doing this, rinse the lentils and add them to a pan of boiling water, and cook until they're completely soft, and slightly 'fluffy' at the edges. Strain the lentils, take the garlic and sweet potato from the oven, and let everything cool before mixing together. Add the lime juice, the remaining olive oil, salt and pepper and coriander/cilantro, and stir together until fully combined. If you prefer a lighter consistency you can add more olive oil or lime juice to thin the dip (it shouldn't be necessary, though).

CAVOLO NERO AND CARROT COLESLAW

Makes 6 portions, with extra mayonnaise for later

Great for late summer to autumn
Suits Pitta and Kapha types

I went years and years without enjoying coleslaw (that horribly fake sweet stuff you get in giant tubs in the supermarket was to blame) – but then I tasted a lovely fresh and seasonal vegan version, made with an organic rice-milk mayo and vibrant white cabbage, and it changed everything. My husband makes this delicious version at home and we nosh it with everything from veggie wraps to falafel. The mayonnaise is made traditionally because I believe if you're going to eat it you shouldn't get it out of a jar. Mustard isn't ideal for Pitta, but it's in relatively small quantities here, and in such cases, it's more than okay to go ahead and enjoy.

2 egg yolks
1 garlic clove, finely chopped
A good dash of cider vinegar
A squeeze of lemon or lime
1 tsp Dijon mustard
100ml/scant ½ cup extra virgin olive oil
180ml/ ¾ cup cold-pressed rapeseed/canola oil
1 head of cavolo nero/Tuscan kale, shredded
4 large carrots, cut into matchsticks
Salt and freshly ground black pepper

The key to this is a fresh and piquant mayonnaise. It takes 15 minutes to make and will produce about half a pint/1¼ cups plus 1 tbsp. Beat the egg yolks until smooth. Add the garlic, cider vinegar and a squeeze of lemon or lime juice. Then add the mustard and salt and a good grind of black pepper. Slowly add the olive oil and rapeseed/canola oil, whisking all the time. Ensure that any oil added is whisked in before adding more, to avoid splitting. When all the oil is added, taste and add further seasoning.

Fill a bowl with the cavolo nero/Tuscan kale and carrots. Keep it crunchy and don't shred the veg too thin. Spoon in the mayonnaise so that the cabbage and carrots are just coated. You will be left with a happy surplus of mayo for the coming days.

Ayurvedic Super Sauces

The Power of the Chutney

I went many, many years without ever once considering adding a dash of 'chutney' to my food. Growing up in England, I was familiar with little other than tomato ketchup, mayonnaise, brown sauce and tartar sauce . . . while, being Turkish, I often dolloped plain yogurt or hummus onto my food if I felt it needed a wet, sour or salty hand. Indian chutneys, however, are a different ball game. They're very highly packed with flavour, but they can also serve to aid digestion, stoke agni and just generally add more 'taste' combinations to a meal, which can take a dish from being 'everyday' to supremely satisfying. The only thing that puts me off the traditional Indian chutneys (particularly shop-bought ones) are the very high levels of refined sugar. A sweet chutney certainly has its place (I've included one sweet and one savoury below) but it's always best to use a less refined sweetener – jaggery is ideal – or to work with the natural sweetness of your ingredients instead, which if good, will still pack a tasty punch.

FENNEL AND CORIANDER CHUTNEY

Great for summer and autumn

Suits all dosha types

1 tbsp ghee

1 large fennel bulb (or 2 small), diced very small

2 spring onions/scallions, very finely diced, or cut into 1mm/⅓in thin rings

2 tbsp fresh coriander/cilantro, chopped

1 tbsp extra virgin olive oil

2 tbsp lime juice

A pinch of salt

A pinch of white pepper

Over a medium heat, add the ghee to a pan, let it melt, then add the fennel and spring onions/scallions, and lightly sauté until they begin to soften. You do not want to 'cook' them, just to take the edge off their rawness. Remove from the heat and let cool. Add the coriander/cilantro, olive oil, lime juice, salt and pepper, and stir everything together well, then transfer into a sterile jar, where this will keep in the refrigerator for 1–2 weeks.

PAPAYA AND LIME CHUTNEY

Great for summer
Suits Vata types; Pitta can eat occasionally

1 tbsp jaggery
1 tsp sea salt
60ml/¼ cup lime juice
Approx 100g/scant 1½ cups papaya, peeled,
    deseeded, finely chopped
40g/¼ cup white onion, finely diced
1 tbsp fresh ginger, finely grated
1 large handful coriander/cilantro, finely chopped
1 tsp fresh chilli, very finely chopped (Pitta types
    should use fresh mint instead, as should anyone
    who doesn't like chilli)

Mix the jaggery and salt in the lime juice until completely
dissolved. Transfer to a bowl and add the papaya, onion, ginger,
coriander/cilantro and chilli, stirring well to combine and soak
in the juice. Serve as it is, or transfer to jars, refrigerate and let
soak for a day or two – the flavour will continue to intensify. This
should store well for up to a month.

POWER GREEN PESTO

Great for all seasons
Suits all dosha types

'Pesto' comes from the Italian 'pestaro', meaning to pound or crush
(this is also where the word pestle, as in pestle and mortar, comes

210

from). We're very used to eating the basil, pine nut and parmesan variety – scan any supermarket shelf and you'll see many versions of this traditional mainstay – but the concept stretches brilliantly. Just as Thai cooks make up the base for their sauces by pounding lemongrass, garlic, chilli, etc., in a mortar, with a pestle, to make their 'paste', Ayurvedic cooks can really benefit from the same approach. This very quick and easy 'pesto' can be eaten with anything – spread on sandwiches, mixed into rice or pasta, used as a marinade, dolloped upon soup . . . It's a great fallback snack as parsley and coriander/cilantro are both tri-doshic, and will balance every dosha, while seriously stoking agni too.

1 small bunch coriander/cilantro leaves and stems,
    with dry/woody bits of the stems cut off
1 small bunch parsley
240ml/1 cup extra virgin olive oil
168g/1 cup flax or pumpkin seeds
1 tsp pink Himalayan salt
Very generous grind of black pepper
Juice of half a fresh lime, squeezed

Put all the ingredients in a blender and whizz up until you get a lovely smooth, even paste. Eat what you want, and scoop the rest into clean sterile jars, seal and refrigerate, where it should keep for up to 2 weeks.

Good, Sweet Snacks

Because I do have a sweet tooth, I've spent a lot of time working out the best ways to keep it in check, without curbing it entirely (I figure, if I enjoy something and I can make it myself from good ingredients, then it's a perfectly legitimate indulgence). Great to make up if you have spare time at the weekend, and pack in work lunchboxes, or have to hand if the sweet munchies strike after dinner!

CHIA CHOC BARS
Makes about 12

Great for all seasons
Suits Vata types; Pitta can eat occasionally

1 tbsp jaggery
30g/¼ cup pumpkin seeds, shelled, raw
4 tbsp whole chia seeds
2 tbsp sunflower seeds
50g/¼ cup dried dates, finely chopped and pitted
  (Kapha should use dried figs instead)
30g/generous ⅓ cup desiccated/dry unsweetened
  coconut
About 160g/2 cups rolled oats
3 tbsp cocoa powder

Preheat the oven to 200°C/400°F/gas mark 6. Lightly grease a 30 x 20cm/12 x 8in baking tin (a 2.2 litre/2 quart rectangular baking tin) with oil and line with baking parchment. In a saucepan set over low heat, melt the coconut oil, then add the maple syrup, sugar and jaggery. When everything is melted, add the pumpkin, chia and sunflower seeds, dates and coconut and stir well, ensuring they're all soaked in the liquid. Then add the oats, handful by handful, stirring the mixture the whole time so that each handful is coated and absorbing the liquid before you add more. Once the oats start to clump together and as you stir they stop soaking up any liquid (or no liquid remains and the mixture feels firm), stop adding oats. Spoon the mixture into the prepared baking tin, packing it down with the back of a wooden spoon. Pop it in the oven for 15–20 minutes, but check the mixture every so often – you want to turn the oven off once it turns a deep golden colour, before it goes brown. Turn the heat off and let it rest in the oven for 10 minutes. Then remove, score with a knife into bars, and let cool. Once cool, you can cut the bars along your scored lines, and place in an airtight container, where they'll last for a week.

SWEET DREAM CHAI

Serves 1

Great for all seasons
Suits all dosha types

It's official – Brits are a bunch of chai latte lovers (did you know that Starbucks sell more of these in the UK than anywhere else in Europe put together?).

If you're one of those people who are addicted to this comforting, sweetly spicy drink, here's a miraculous health-boosting recipe to try at home. Fennel seeds aid digestion, cardamom boosts immunity, cloves contain eugenol, which is similar to dopamine in its ability to help the body relax, and almond milk is naturally cholesterol-free and boosts metabolism. Talk about a dream drink! Almond milk tastes naturally sweet, but if the mixture in the pan is not sweet enough for your palate, Vata and Pitta types can try stirring in a teaspoon of honey, maple syrup or jaggery once the milk has cooled down a bit.

225ml/scant 1 cup almond milk (or soy milk
   for Kapha)
2 cardamom pods
½ tsp fennel seeds
3 cloves

Put all the ingredients in a pan and bring to the boil. Remove from heat and allow to steep for 3 minutes. Pour through a strainer into your favourite mug.

COCOA NIB AND COCONUT GRANOLA

Serves 6 generously

Great for autumn and winter
Suits Vata and Pitta types

I use this in lots of ways. It's great with nut milk for breakfast and blends well with other cereals, such as cornflakes or bran flakes, so

214

you can use it to amp up the flavour and texture of a cereal you're a bit bored of. It's also a delicious topping for a crumble, and an extra crunchy treat atop some good coconut yoghurt or vanilla ice cream.

50g/¼ cup coconut oil
3 tbsp maple syrup
1 tbsp jaggery
180g/scant 2¼ cups porridge/rolled oats
80g/1 cup desiccated/dry unsweetened coconut
1 tbsp cocoa nibs

Preheat the oven to 190°C/375°F/gas mark 5. Melt the coconut oil in a pan. Add the maple syrup and jaggery and stir through. Add the oats, coconut and cocoa nibs and stir into the liquid, ensuring that all the oats get a good coating of the liquid. Tip out onto a 32 x 22cm/13 x 9in baking tray/cookie sheet, lined and greased, and shake to spread evenly. Toast in the oven for 10–12 minutes, until golden brown. Leave to cool, then store in an airtight container, where it should last for up to 2 weeks.

BAKED APRICOTS

Serves 5

Great for summer
Suits all doshas

Apricots are a lovely tri-doshic fruit, so it's nice to take advantage of something that everyone can eat! Although Ayurveda advises eating fruit on an empty stomach, if you do have an early light dinner and fancy dessert a couple of hours later – or even better, something sweet after lunch – you can't go far wrong with this fragrant treat. You want your apricots to be ripe but still have firmness, otherwise they'll disintegrate too much when you cook them.

10 small ripe organic apricots, washed, pitted
   and halved
5 cinnamon sticks (also known as cassia bark)
20 cloves
Maple syrup, for drizzling

Preheat the oven to 180°C/350°F/gas mark 4. Place the apricots skin side down, evenly spaced, in a baking tin. Break the cinnamon sticks in half. Drizzle syrup over each apricot, then stick a clove into each one and place the cinnamon evenly across the tin, so that each apricot is in contact with both a clove and a piece of cinnamon. Pop into the oven and bake for 15 minutes, or until the apricots start to caramelize and are lovely and soft. Once cool, remove the cinnamon and cloves.

FURTHER READING
AND RESOURCES

Reading List

Lad, Usha and Vasant Usha, *Ayurvedic Cooking for Self-Healing*, 2nd edn, Ayurvedic Press, Albuquerque, 2002

Lad, Vasant, *Ayurveda: The Science of Self-Healing*, Lotus Press, Santa Fe, 1984

Morningstar, Amadea with Urmila Desai, *The Ayurvedic Cookbook*, Lotus Press, Santa Fe, 1990

Pole, Sebastian, *A Pukka Life*, Quadrille, London, 2011. A hugely informative and entertaining read – a vast rich wealth of information that you'll keep referring back to. Great on all things seasonal too.

Svoboda, Robert E, *Ayurveda: Life, Health and Longevity*, Ayurvedic Press, Albuquerque, 1992

Svoboda, Robert E, *The Hidden Secret of Ayurveda*, Ayurvedic Press, Albuquerque, 1980

Online Resources

If you're looking to find a reputable Ayurvedic practitioner in the UK, it is a good idea to start with the Ayurvedic Practitioners Association (APA) website – www.apa.uk.com. If you are in the US, visit the National Ayurvedic Medical Association at www.ayurvedanama.org.

www.balanceplan.co.uk is the official website of The Balance Plan. This information-packed lifestyle site is filled with all you need to know to achieve balance in your mind, body and spirit. From online breath, meditation and yoga classes to regularly updated recipes that will make your mouth water (and optimize agni!), this site is aimed at those who need to de-stress, renew, revitalize and rediscover their body's happy, balanced centre. Take the Dosha questionnaire, forward to friends, and begin your journey with wonderful, honest advice and support from The Balance Plan team.

The site also features fantastic tips and interviews with the world's leading health and wellbeing experts, and insights into creating a happy, balanced space within head and home. Sign up for exclusive offers, news and forthcoming events, and the information-packed Balance Mail, a seasonal e-zine that delivers essential support before the seasons change, to ensure you're one step ahead of your health.

www.ayurveda.com offers online learning, training, clinic consultations, recipe ideas and in-depth information on everything about Ayurveda.

Many of the experts I've featured in the book have marvellous resource-filled websites, and logging on is a great way not only to read up on wellbeing issues, but also to hear news of special offers and upcoming events. These websites can also be a great source of good-quality supplies, such as Ayurvedic herbs, supplements and body oils.

www.consciousfood.co.uk – suppliers of organic food and nutraceuticals, including the Conscious Food D'Mix, a natural remedy for digestive gas.

www.demamiel.com – the de Mamiel and Botaniques ranges of natural, organic skincare, from Annee de Mamiel.

www.evekalinik.com – nutritional advice from Eve Kalinik.

www.movementformodernlife.com – easy yoga classes offered online, in 10-, 20- or 30-minute segments, to fit into even the busiest lives.

www.powerfulyoga.co.uk – website of yoga teacher Selda Enver Goodwin.

www.pukkaherbs.com – brand-leaders in the production of exceptional-quality Ayurvedic herbs; they sell a great Triphala.

www.sustainweb.org/realbread – campaigning for better bread.

www.theorganicpharmacy.com – offers organic skincare, make-up and perfume, as well as supplements and homeopathic remedies. They provide beauty and health treatments through their stores and spa partners around the world. Try the detox programme outlined in a fact sheet on the website.

www.tri-dosha.co.uk – resources for living Ayurvedically, including Ayurvedic skincare and bodycare products, consultations and retreats, recommendations for holistic suppliers, and a blog.

Recommended Supplements

For your daily probiotic, I favour Viridian, Symprove, Udo's Choice, the Organic Pharmacy and Bio-Kult varieties (all available at health food stores or online).

A good combined enzyme taken daily in capsule form helps with food digestion. Brands I have tried and liked include Atone, Biocare and Udo's Choice.

The Conscious Food D'Mix is a blend of herbs and spices to chew after meals to aid digestion. I have found it much more effective in relieving gas than chemist/drugstore alternatives such as Wind-eze.

I am also a big fan of Udo's Choice Ultimate Oil, which provides a wonderfully balanced blend of omega 3, 6 and 9 oils to ensure the right amount of essential fats within the body.

Fun and Inspiring Blogs

www.food-alovestory.com – a friendly and engaging site, with some great Ayurveda-inspired recipes.

www.joyfullbelly.com – an enormous catalogue of information: primarily recipes posted by the active Ayurvedic community of this site. A great browsing ground.

www.wholesomelovinggoodness.com – a positive and happiness-filled blog that shares wonderful recipes and simple advice, via lovely Lorien, who lives in Australia.

INDEX

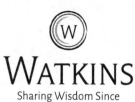

WATKINS

Sharing Wisdom Since
1893

The story of Watkins Publishing dates back to March 1893, when John M. Watkins, a scholar of esotericism, overheard his friend and teacher Madame Blavatsky lamenting the fact that there was nowhere in London to buy books on mysticism, occultism or metaphysics. At that moment Watkins was born, soon to become the home of many of the leading lights of spiritual literature, including Carl Jung, Rudolf Steiner, Alice Bailey and Chögyam Trungpa.

Today our passion for vigorous questioning is still resolute. With over 350 titles on our list, Watkins Publishing reflects the development of spiritual thinking and new science over the past 120 years. We remain at the cutting edge, committed to publishing books that change lives.

DISCOVER MORE ...

Read our blog

Watch and listen to
our authors in action

Sign up to
our mailing list

JOIN IN THE CONVERSATION

WatkinsPublishing   @watkinswisdom

WatkinsPublishingLtd   +watkinspublishing1893

Our books celebrate conscious, passionate, wise and happy living.
Be part of the community by visiting

www.watkinspublishing.com